Hospice and Palliative Care
an interdisciplinary approach

edited by

Dame Cicely Saunders OM, DBE, FRCP
Founder of St. Christopher's Hospice, London

Edward Arnold
A division of Hodder & Stoughton
LONDON MELBOURNE AUCKLAND

© 1990 Cicely Saunders

First published in Great Britain 1990
Reprinted 1991 (with corrections)

British Library Cataloguing in Publication Data
Saunders, Dame, Cicely
   Hospice and palliative care : an interdisciplinary approach.
   1. Terminally ill patients. Care
   362.175

   ISBN 0-340-54462-7

Typeset in 11/12pt Palatino by
Hewer Text Composition Services, Edinburgh
Printed and bound in Great Britain for Edward Arnold,
a division of Hodder and Stoughton Limited,
Mill Road, Dunton Green, Sevenoaks, Kent TN13 2YA by
Biddles Ltd, Guildford and King's Lynn

Contents

Contributors List

Mary J. Baines, MB, BChir. Consultant Physician

Helene Channon, RGN. Ward Sister

Margaret Harris, B.Ed (Hons. Cantab), RGN. Chaplain's Assistant

Linda Jackson, RGN. Ward Sister

Len Lunn, Revd. Chaplain

Barbara Monroe, BA, B.Phil., CQSW. Director of Social Work

Marie Murphy, MRCPI. Senior Registrar

Tony O'Brien, MRCPI. Consultant Physician

Betty O'Gorman, MCSP, SRP. Superintendent Physiotherapist

Barbara Saunders, FRCN. Director of Nursing

Cicely Saunders, OM, DBE, FRCP. Chairman

Alison Virdee, RGN. Ward Sister

Tom West, OBE, MB, BS. Medical Director

Bridget Wood, MRGP. Registrar

All from St. Christopher's Hospice, London

Introduction

Over 60 years ago Peabody wrote, 'The secret of the care of the patient is in caring for the patient' (Peabody, 1927). This aphorism sums up the philosophy that lies behind the method of working we have tried to describe in this book. In the same paper he also wrote, 'What is spoken of as a "clinical picture" is not just a photograph of a man sick in bed; it is an impressionistic picture of the patient surrounded by his home, his work, his relations, his friends, his joys, sorrows, hopes and fears' (Peabody, 1927).

It is this scene that we are addressing and, in our turn, we do so as another composite picture. We are, as it were, a collage comprised of all the different professions involved in the total care of the person who is approaching death. In the home the 'artist' will be the leader of the primary health care team; in a hospital or hospice ward it may well be the ward sister who builds the picture together in the management of the team, while the leadership in addressing a specific problem, be it clinical or psychosocial, may finally lie elsewhere. This is addressed by Dr. West in his chapter on *Principles* as he sets the scene and by Sister Jackson as she turns to its practicalities in a ward.

We have to put together our basic philosophy of inter-disciplinary working in the setting of the four separate wards and Home Care Team of a teaching and training hospice. We have looked at some of the mechanics of building these teams together in a hospice where the average in-patient stay is some three weeks and many of the staff come for a limited time for a training programme. The great majority of our patients will die with us, often after more than one admission for symptom control and after a time at home with the support of our team there added to the main community resources. They are a group referred with problems that others believe need specialized care. Although other problems may be part of a complex presentation, pain is the major symptom that brings patients to us and a multi-professional approach to this 'total pain' is almost always called for as we face its emotional, social and spiritual elements to compound the physical. This, of course, is also the approach of the multi-professional Pain Clinic but in our field there is the added pressure of limited time and often urgent demands for reconciliations and farewells. Dr. Baines' pivotal chapter addresses this before we turn to a series of other challenges. The Hospice or Support or Palliative Care Team has to move fast and with smooth communication if patient and family strengths and peace are to be found. We hope the urgency and pressure of time that we face together will make the approach we have set out to describe relevant to readers in other settings but will also bring the clarity of a concentrated focus. Any crisis can identify priorities and enable the participants to move with unexpected speed. Time given at this point may well avoid the call for much more time later.

The second half of the book is a selection of the situations that may occur in any home, clinic or ward, which present both opportunities to grasp and, all too often, arouse deep feelings of failure. They are titles chosen by a 'brainstorming' multi-professional group to present a series of occasions when the team approach is essential if any resolution is to be found. The members are experienced in working, learning and reviewing their work together and they chose these titles to probe their expertise in a demanding and rewarding way. Each contributor has undertaken the responsibility for discussing their chapter with those of other professions with whom they normally work and share problems, so that each writer speaks for more than his or her own discipline and as a team member. Some chapters have been discussed with a large team meeting, others by a few chosen members from the group with whom they normally work and often struggle to find solutions.

All would agree that the people we are trying to help are in a sense also part of the team, at home carrying the main burden of care and always involved wherever the patient may be. This of course is especially true in the care of the children of a dying parent or grandparent. Here they are the most important carers and communicators. At other times it is perhaps unrealistic in many situations to term them the leaders of the team but there is no doubt that it is they who, consciously or not, are the ones to set the agenda. Peabody put his patient in the centre of his impressionistic picture; the interdisciplinary team, while keeping the same focus, tries to give attention to every aspect of the whole scene.

Although we have included specific suggestions in a few areas, this is not primarily intended as a 'how to' book. The investigations and treatments that enable much of the patient and family interchange are covered well elsewhere. Rather it is a sharing of what has grown over the past 22 years into a challenging and supportive way of working in an often demanding field, as we have learnt not only to work together but also when and how to call in and co-operate with consultants of various specialities and with other teams. We hope that this is ready now to fill a gap in the literature and to be shared with all those who aim to enhance the quality of living and of relationships for their patients and families when there is only a limited time left.

Cicely Saunders
1990

Reference

PEABODY F. W. (1927). The Care of the Patient. *The Journal of the American Medical Association*, **88**, No. 12, 877–882.

Further Reading

AINSWORTH-SMITH, I., and SPECK, P. (1982). *Letting Go*. SPCK, London.

BUCKMAN, R. (1988). *I Don't Know What to Say: How to help and support someone who is dying*. Papermac, London.

DUNLOP, R. J., and HOCKLEY, J. M. (1990). *Terminal Care Support Teams – The Hospital/Hospice Interface*. Oxford University Press, Oxford.

NEUBERGER, J. (1987). *Caring for People of Different Faiths*. Austen Cornish Publishers in association with The Lisa Sainsbury Foundation, London.

SAUNDERS, C. (Ed.) (1984) *The Management of Terminal Malignant Disease* (2nd Edn). Edward Arnold, London.

SAUNDERS, C. and BAINES, M. (1989) *Living with Dying: the management of terminal disease* (2nd Edn). Oxford University Press, Oxford.

STEDEFORD, A. (1984) *Facing Death*. Heinemann.

TWYCROSS, R. G. and LACK, S. A. (1990) *Therapeutics in Terminal Cancer* (2nd Edn). Churchill Livingstone, London and New York.

WALSH, T. D. (1989) *Symptom Control*. Blackwell Scientific Publications, London and Boston.

WORLD HEALTH ORGANISATION (1986) *Cancer Pain Relief*. World Health Organisation, Geneva.

PART I

Principles of Interdisciplinary Work in Hospice and Palliative Care

1

Multidisciplinary Working

Tom West

Introduction

Helping people with far advanced cancer calls for more
skills than any one individual can command. The inter-
disciplinary team approach has been developed in
disciplines such as paediatrics where the whole family
needs to be involved. Nowhere is it more essential than
in response to the expressed and perceived needs of
patients in the terminal stages of cancer and also of their
families.

The original concept of the 'total pain' of patients, with
its physical, psycho-social and spiritual components has
now been enlarged to include staff involvement and
stress together with all the pains that this can arouse. At
the same time the importance of 'family' in the widest
sense of the word, present or absent (and even alive or
dead) is seen as an area to be explored and one in which
there are often hidden strengths to be uncovered in
otherwise impossible situations. Furthermore, working
in this way does not have to be confined to independent,
free standing hospices. It can also be appropriate in
caring for patients at home, in hospitals and in nursing

homes, each of which has its own advantages and dis-
advantages.

Selection

The interdisciplinary team is formed from a group of
individuals who will undoubtedly have been drawn to this
work for a variety of reasons. Most care-givers have
personal reasons for needing to care, and a wish to understand and be involved in the dynamics of patient and family
as well as in team work is a good beginning. A successful
working team must begin with careful selection: professional
competence, flexibility, a sense of humour, respect for
others, the ability to support colleagues and above all an
awareness of what is meant by trust are all needed.

There are as many selection procedures as there are
institutions and it is hard to strike a balance between a
democratic approach in which everyone has to be involved,
and an autocratic appointment, which if less than a total
success can be expected to bring with it much resentment. A
clear idea by those interviewing as well as by the candidate,
of the common task and therefore of the accepted objectives,
is a good base-line for the interview. Some discussion of
shared beliefs and therefore of the possibility of disagree-
ment is important because in spite of possessing the highest
professional skills, team members may sometimes be asked
to modify professional practice and the acceptability (or
otherwise) of this should be explored.

Following the appointment a trial period is essential and
from the beginning, needs to be recognised as a two-way
exercise. During it there must be regular occasions for
appraisal between the new team member and the team
leader and both here and on into longer term team
functioning there must be opportunities for growth that are
not just patient centred. Although patient and family are
the reason for the existence of the team and therefore for
the presence of the individuals who make up the team,
it is essential that team members can on occasions deal

directly with each other, learning and developing in the process.

The Team

In interdisciplinary work responsibility is shared. Each member of the team brings to the day's work his or her own professional skills with all the confidence that this produces. But professional traditions will also be present and may well need adjusting. The stereotype of each profession (e.g. doctor, nurse, social worker) can be almost as easily imposed as assumed. Each team member may also have to deal with personal stereotyping and work out with the team how such type-casting is best used or, if necessary, overcome.

This involves looking for and beginning to understand the professional and personal skills of other disciplines as well as one's own, recognizing the fact of professional rivalries and the temptation to compete, and learning how to share and when to hand over. It is not natural to be generous, to share the particular gifts or skills that mark one out, nor is it easy to be prepared to give up being 'the one' to complete a fine piece of work. But the symbolism and the effectiveness of professions working jointly, yet able at times to appear to abdicate roles without loss of face, is one of the major strengths of the interdisciplinary approach. The doctor who is able to step aside for the social worker and the nurse who knows when she does *not* need to call the chaplain represent effective functioning by all four of these different disciplines.

Team Functions

In practice no team can afford to be leader-less, but there is an important if less than clear distinction between the leader and the manager of an interdisciplinary team. If the team is to continue to function properly decisions have to be taken and this means that every member of the team must have some ideas about necessary boundaries and also about where, if things go wrong, the buck actually stops.

The decision maker may well vary depending on the problem being addressed. In clinical decision-making, for example, it must be the doctor who has the final responsibility. In other words who the leader or key worker or current 'worrier' is should depend on the nature of the problem being faced. The rest of the team will, of course, be available for appropriate discussion and consultation.

But at the same time if the work is to continue and not just rock from crisis to crisis there must be a manager to ensure day to day continuity. For example on a hospice or hospital ward, the ward sister (rather than the doctor) is the obvious manager, while in a family meeting the social worker may be the appropriate leader.

A team should be willing to contact and link up with other professional care-givers. For example details of the patient's previous investigations and medical or surgical treatments may need clarifying and here the team doctor should contact the hospital doctor or the general practitioner. If more information about the nursing care of the patient is required it is best obtained by the team nurse from the ward or district nurse who has been looking after the patient. Complicated social problems, perhaps involving confidentiality, will most appropriately be communicated from social worker to social worker.

A team must always be quick to recognise the possible importance of calling on relevant outside help. Radiotherapists, oncologists, anaesthetists and surgeons may still have something to offer even towards the end of a patient's life. Involving the available community services may enable a patient to stay at home for longer and may support the family through a time of otherwise overwhelming stress. Clearly deciding who in the team should be responsible for making such contacts and for ensuring that things run smoothly is part of the overall management needed if everything that ought to be done for the patient and his family is to be achieved.

A team will need a sense of purpose and vision. The source is often hard to identify. Where good management has provided a safe enough context anyone in the team may feel able to propose a change of plan, confident that they will be listened to with respect and then supported in their individual or collective actions. Such a team will find that it has the strength to admit mistakes and change direction without scape-goating. All this will depend on a clear but flexible organisation and an acknowledgement of who, when the chips are down, has the last word.

Organisation and Communication

Recognizing who is leading and respecting who is quietly managing is the bare bones of a system that forms the basis of good interdisciplinary work.

But decisions must not only be made, they must also be communicated and recorded and they will still need reviewing.

Working with patients suffering from advanced disease demands not just tender loving care – there must also be skilful loving care and there will often be a need for quick decisions and quick communication. In practice it is often impossible for everyone to be informed of everything and this necessary limitation of the numbers involved calls for an exercise in trust by those who would otherwise feel excluded.

At the same time this work necessitates enough time and enough staff for there to be effective day to day hand-overs. Good reporting from one shift to another should be treated as a priority. For example following a family meeting during the day no night staff should have to work through the night without appropriate knowledge of what went on. The next day is too late. For less urgent matters the most economical occasion for communication is the inter-disciplinary weekly team meeting. When these are well managed and well led the level of communication is amazingly high and the sources of information often surprising. It may be the physiotherapist who supplies the missing link in a problem situation. Perhaps the confidence shared with the physiotherapist has occurred because the doctor is the doctor, nurses work in pairs and social workers do not wear uniforms. It is the one to one, hands-on meeting with an obvious 'professional' that encourages the patient to talk.

There are guidelines for interdisciplinary meetings that can be helpful: the right language for communication at these meetings must be learned. Professional jargon even to other professionals is counter-productive. A room is needed that is comfortable enough, private enough and the right shape for easy communication. Bleeps should, if possible, be left outside. At such weekly meetings teams will slowly learn more about getting it right, as they go through match re-plays of both successes and failures, and look at the detail and the timing of personal interventions just as carefully as they plan the pharmacological ones.

Communicating with and advising professionals outside the team is a further skill to be mastered. Discussing the pros and cons of further active therapy with an oncologist or giving advice about drugs to a general practitioner is not always straightforward. With practise, and as each side gets to know the other better, it becomes easier. Taking the trouble to meet the other person on his or her own ground or inviting them to visit the hospice or palliative care unit can transform an otherwise difficult situation.

Other Important Team Activities

There are other important priorities in the life of a team.

Ward rounds
should be fixed points in the week's programme. It is useful if an interdisciplinary discussion can take place before the patients are visited. Here the manager – usually the senior nurse – can bring the other disciplines up to date with

patients and their families; fore-warned can be fore-armed. Possible changes in treatment should be discussed and provisional plans of action proposed.

Who visits the bed-side depends on both availability and appropriateness. Three or four people are usually the maximum that can sit round a bed without it feeling oppressive. Here it is usual for the doctor to be leader while the senior nurse or the social worker may well be cast in the role of patient's advocate. During discussion it is important that while any two are engaged in conversation the others are observing reactions on both sides and picking up clues as to what is really being said and understood. People round the bed can be drawn into the conversation to help prevent any feeling of an unequal duel between patient and doctor and it is particularly satisfactory if the patient (or sometimes a family member) ends up by taking a leading part in the discussion.

When the ward round is completed team members must take time to go over what has occurred and what they observed. Plans of action can now be confirmed or altered. Decisions will then be recorded.

Of course it is important that team members also do rounds alone, giving the patient the opportunity for a more private interview or a thorough physical examination. But it is essential that such solo visits are fully reported on to the staff responsible for the ongoing management of the ward.

Home visits
may often have to be carried out by a single member of the team. Again as much knowledge as possible should be gathered beforehand from those already involved. It is useful if a check list of the current problems has been drawn up so that these can be checked out and proposals for dealing with them formulated. The visit itself takes place on the patient's territory and it is worth remembering that good manners are as important here as they are at the hospital bed-side. Reporting and recording is vital if continuity of care from one visit to the next is to be maintained by the

team and links with the wider interdisciplinary community services are to be forged and strengthened.

Family meetings

are sometimes anticipated with a degree of fear by team members. Doctors in particular have often had little experience of facing an angry family except perhaps when protected by a white coat or a large desk.

A brief team-meeting beforehand is essential. The strengths as well as the weaknesses of the family should be rehearsed. The objectives of the meeting can be decided on and a provisional agenda and seating plan proposed. If the family concern is primarily medical the doctor will take the initiative. At other times it will be the social worker or the team member closest to the family who starts off as leader, but often a family member rapidly takes over as the spokes-person for the whole group and not infrequently it is the youngest person present who asks the question no one else has the courage to voice.

Perhaps at no other time is the interdisciplinary team approach more obviously appropriate. The family will see the team's wide-ranging concern for their needs while, at the same time, they experience a model of different people trying to work together in ways that can often be usefully applied to their own situation. Recording such meetings while respecting confidentiality can be difficult, but again it is important that team members not present are informed of matters that have arisen and are relevant to their ongoing care of the family.

Assessment visits

are a special skill. Those carrying them out must have real experience of the possible course and problems of the disease. They also need to be aware of the current strengths and weaknesses both of the team and of the institution they represent. It is irresponsible to accept a patient or family that the team, for whatever reason, is not able to care for appropriately.

Other Matters

Reporting and Confidentiality

If the interdisciplinary team is to function reasonably smoothly then reports, recording and handovers have to be conducted efficiently. It is not always easy to distinguish what is relevant and important from what is routine trivia. When matters of confidentiality are involved it must be accepted that not everyone has to know everything. Indeed no one needs to know more than will enable them to fulfil their own role in caring for the patient. If a patient chooses to unburden personal matters to a member of the team it can be very helpful to say something like: 'Thank you for sharing such an important and difficult thing with me. Would you mind if in turn I shared it with other members of the team?' Almost always the person, pleased to be the centre of such real concern, will agree.

Teaching

An important function of the interdisciplinary team should be to teach. Sometimes this may feel like an unwanted and heavy load but in fact it can be both stimulating and a first-class antidote to battle-fatigue. Teaching other people what is on offer and how best to use the team and its individual members obviously makes good sense. Experience will then help to show them when the team's skills really should be called on, when team involvement is quite unnecessary or when all that is needed is back-up from the team.

But teaching non-team members appropriate skills in hospice and palliative care will only succeed if they are also given sufficient confidence in their ability to take on these rather wider roles. Nothing succeeds better in building confidence than giving appropriate praise. Nothing is more destructive than public criticism.

Other Questions

There will always be further questions for a team to address if it wishes to continue to develop:

- What makes people tired? Genuine pressure of work, ill-health, personal problems, battles with administration, communication problems, inadequate resources, unrealistic expectations are some of the factors that a tired team (or a team with a tired team-member) would be wise to explore.
- How does a team take on a new member? Marriages may be made in heaven, they certainly have to be worked at on earth. Taking the trouble to make space for the newcomer can help turn what feels in the first place an intruder into a valued addition to the team.
- How does a team cope when they are short staffed and there is still a mountain of work that has to be done? It is extraordinarily difficult to lower standards or to cut corners, yet the real choice may end up between leaving work undone or, for the emergency, to work faster.

Summary

The interdisciplinary team has to look outside itself and recognize and learn how and when it is appropriate to incorporate different disciplines. Occupational Therapy and the other important therapies, volunteers, the administrative staff all have vital roles to play. Too often lip service is paid to their supportive membership of the team, when in practice not enough care has been taken in first carefully defining their special function and then appropriately including them in.

The interdisciplinary team approach is an exercise in learning, caring, working together, teaching and appraisal.

It cannot succeed without enough individual professional skill and enough trust and understanding between the professions to give each member the courage to follow his own judgement when that is what seems appropriate. Taking such considered risks is often only possible with the knowledge that the team is providing a solid stage for actions than can lead to a positive approach and real creativity in otherwise overwhelming problems.

Team work is often more untidy than tidy – so is the rest of life. But honest reviewing by the team of the work as it proceeds will usually result in a sense of job satisfaction rather than one of despondency. And just because it is not possible to take on new commitments when there is too much unfinished business still in hand, the occasions taken by a team to affirm achievements and to acknowledge the ending of successive pieces of work is good use of their time.

Finally, it is difficult to overrate the importance of appropriate praise and a respect for such phrases as 'Good morning', 'Thank you' and occasionally, 'I was wrong, I'm sorry'. Good manners can enable a team to get through times of mis-understanding and also to cash in successfully on crisis situations when, just by *not* playing it safe, often the impossible is achieved.

2

Team Building

Linda Jackson

The complex demands of palliative care cannot be adequately met through the isolated strivings of individual health care workers. It is suggested that the essence of hospice care is teamwork (Manning, 1984). However, teams do not necessarily function just because they exist. If you place a heterogeneous group of people together and call them a 'team', this does not ensure an effective collaboration of workers. A team is not a static entity and teamwork is a continuous process. Therefore this chapter attempts to define the nature of a team, characteristics of a successful team and suggests how team building and maintenance may be facilitated. As a ward sister my experience of team building is in that setting and will be biased towards this area but the principles may be applicable to any group of people trying to work together in any field.

Attributes of the Successful Working Team

A team is a group of persons with a common purpose working together. For a group of people to work as a team and not as individuals there needs to be a team spirit – a willingness to act for the benefit of one's group rather than oneself; an esprit de corps. This team spirit engenders team work – a combined effort which demonstrates the art of cooperation. It is pertinent to discuss the attributes of a successful team in order to understand what one is trying to build and maintain. There appear to be four main elements in the functioning team: group purpose, role definition, communication and leadership. The team leader provides the environment in which the team can build itself. It is for this reason that the leader is the vital component of the successful team and this will be addressed in the section 'Maintaining the Team.'

A prerequisite for a functioning team is for each team member to have an understanding of the common goal and his unique role and contribution in its accomplishment. An underlying premise is that no individual possesses all the expertise necessary for the task in hand (i.e. care of the patient and his family), but that the team is committed to the sharing of responsibilities and skills for the patients. Teamwork is a partnership of equals; however, the most salient need of a patient at a given time may give one role precedence. Each team member is competent in his professional capacity and is orientated to and respectful of the professional role and contribution of fellow team members. Team membership is a dynamic entity, roles may change and develop with a changing situation. A good team has members who are able to exhibit maturity in their flexibility and adaptability; recognising their own primary area of responsibility but simultaneously being alert to other areas of patient need. Clear definitions of group purpose and roles within the team are essential.

The strength of the interdisciplinary (ID) team approach is in the diversity of talent which it brings to the task; its vulnerability lies in its necessity for coordination (Zimmerman, 1981). Coordination is essential for the smooth functioning of a team and requires both good communication and good leadership. Without clear channels of communication cooperation becomes impossible. Failing communication in a team is analogous to a failing circulatory system caused by atherosclerosis; it will lead to a painful decrease in the effectiveness of the team and ultimately to its premature death. Within good communication are characteristics of openness, honesty (with tact), an observant sensitivity to the needs of others and a mutual trust enabling a sharing of vulnerabilities as well as strengths. Communication in a functioning team is free in both the vertical plane (giving and receiving of orders) and in the horizontal plane (between team members).

A good team is egalitarian; it avoids cliques, is inclusive of all its members, is welcoming to new members and fosters feelings of belonging. A surviving team is one which maintains a climate of mutual support for stress management in this demanding field of work.

Building the Team

Having described some of the attributes of a successful working team, how does one achieve this utopian state? There is no text book of team building, no 'DIY' manual which if followed will guarantee the desired result. The nature of a team, comprising a dynamic population of individual human beings who each respond to environmental stimuli in a different way, is such that each team will be different and there is no fail-safe prescription for success. Thus what follows is not dogma but some guidelines which may be useful. Perhaps one may consider team building in two parts, namely creating the team and maintaining the team, as there are different elements in both.

1. Creating the Team

There are two important areas for consideration when founding a team: a philosophy of care and staff selection.

Team Philosophy

A unified approach is essential for a successful team. A team begins as a group of individuals and needs common ground to build upon. It is useful to determine a philosophy of care; this is usually a concise statement of the attitudes, values and beliefs about issues which are considered important. Thus, when establishing a team, formulating a philosophy of care may provide direction and a premise from which to work. Individuals bring their own beliefs and ideas to their work and without a commitment to the philosophy of the team they join, all sense of direction will be lost with disharmony the inevitable result. If the organisation's principles are made clear at the outset then one can ensure that all who subsequently join the team are able to work comfortably according to those principles. A philosophy of care may be said to provide a conceptual framework for practice.

Staff Selection

A team leader, however good, is ultimately dependent on the willingness and motivation of the team to ensure its smooth running. In the ideal team there will be a complementary mix of personalities and skills but in reality there will be varying degrees of commitment and 'difficult' and 'unpopular' team members, so consideration to staff selection is important to the building of a team. Qualities to be sought in a potential team member include professional competence which provides a firm basis for respect from colleagues, and an ability to communicate well. Effective communication within a team needs to be two-way, members should be able to listen and speak. It cannot be overemphasized that communication is the lifeline of the team and if team members are poor communicators then difficulties can be anticipated from the outset. A good team member needs to relate well to colleagues, be sensitive to their needs and should express a desire and commitment to team work over and above self-interest. They should also exhibit flexibility and adaptability – a rigid individual may hamper the development of a dynamic team, especially in terminal care where rapidly changing situations sometimes demand a change in role. There needs to be demonstrated maturity in a readiness to be open to others, allowing them to step into a situation and take over if the need arises. These characteristics should be sought on application forms and at interview. The process of staff selection may also be aided by an induction period during which both parties may assess the suitability of the applicant and after which a formal appointment is made.

2. Maintaining the Team

It is unrealistic to presume that a team once formed will be successfully self-perpetuating. As a building requires maintenance work for the upkeep of its fabric, so a team requires continued input to keep it functioning effectively and to maintain its integrity. Commitment to a team means commitment to its growth and development, and this requires effort. One can look at maintaining a team under the four areas identified earlier.

Group Purpose

It has been suggested that each team member should be aware of the direction and purpose of the team and its philosophy. For this to happen the philosophy should be available and offered to new team members and, as a refresher, to existing members. In conjunction with a printed document, a sense of direction may be maintained by open discussion and constant evaluation. As the composition of a team alters, so the agreement with, commitment to and clarity of the team philosophy may change. Thus it may be helpful periodically to discuss these issues, to ask the team to evaluate their achievements and to redefine their aims if necessary. A team is dynamic; recognition of this may aid continuing development of the team in response to the changing pressures in palliative care. A team needs constant updating; a team drifting aimlessly towards unspoken, nebulous goals can create insecurity and dissatisfaction. It is crucial that the goals are realistic.

Role Definition

As it is essential to have clear role definition when establishing a team it is also useful to continue discussion periodically to increase awareness of it. Asking team members to define their role and then to compare and contrast their definition with that of the team leader and other team members may be beneficial. Discussion of each other's role within a team enables mutual expectations to be voiced and may enable role expansion.

Communication

Facilitation of effective communication in the team is vital to its success. From experience, a key element is the allocation of time in which communication may occur. In palliative care, demands on staff are enormous and it is all too easy to be too busy to stop and communicate effectively. Communication may be on a one to one level or amongst the whole group; both are important to the life of the team. One to one communication is easier to arrange providing attention is paid to the need for privacy. A regular time set aside to meet is vital for the life of the whole team. A time especially allocated for group meetings helps to stress the importance of communicating and reduces feelings of guilt about time spent in such meetings. The group meeting is the ideal medium for the dissemination of information relating to work, the sharing of new ideas, discussion of difficult problems, support and for joint evaluation of the team's performance.

In our experience it has been useful for the ID team to meet once a week. This is a regular set time, with a defined length, enabling people to plan their timetables accordingly; it is important to be inclusive of all staff. These meetings are not solely a vehicle for discussing patients but they present an ideal opportunity for sharing expertise, experiences and occasionally perhaps failings. Within the group meeting the leader can try to effect quality time by attention to some ground rules. There needs to be a chairperson (not necessarily the team leader) who should define at the outset of the meeting the length and aim of the meeting, ensuring that this agenda and time schedule are adhered to.

The purpose of the meeting is best served when everyone feels safe enough to contribute. How are these meetings made safe? A central theme in this area is effective communication. A group of people may sit in a room and talk but may not be communicating in any sense. Communication takes place on more than one level; it is not just the dissemination of information about the team's work. The multitude of problems and emotive issues which may be raised when caring for the dying patient and his family need to be shared with the team. Recognition of the importance of feelings of individuals, and permission to discuss them helps to maintain the health of both the individual and the team. However, for good communication in this area to take place people need to learn to take risks with each other. In order to do this individuals need to feel secure and valued within the team. This knowledge of self-worth and contribution to the team may be encouraged through praise and feedback. In a team where everyone seems to be an expert in their own field it can be very threatening to talk about personal feelings. An atmosphere is required in which there is no hidden agenda, so that people can make statements in the knowledge that they will be accepted at face value. It is vital in a team to be able to admit 'I find this situation very hard' or 'I just don't know what to say to Mr. X.'. Team members need to feel comfortable with their colleagues and know that they are respected. A good team is able to accept the weaknesses as well as the strengths of each member, recognising its own frailties and learning from others. How vital for a team of 'experts' to acknowledge their humanity.

Within the ID team it is important that vital information is received at the right time and not heard 'on the grape vine'. Communication in nursing teams regularly takes place by means of the shift handovers. Again, effective communication needs to be stressed here, as often too much irrelevant information is imparted. An attempt to rationalise what is communicated may reduce time wasted on unhelpful issues (e.g. whether Mr X had a bath or a wash) and create time for other discussions and staff support.

The Team Leader

The team leader plays a vital role in all areas of team building and is discussed in this section for the sake of simplicity, but it is recognised as important in the other areas.

The team leader could be viewed as a 'signpost' – visible and directing people. However, the team leader is not the ultimate information carrier but knows who in her team can best inform at any given time. She is aware of what the team is doing and encourages its input rather than her own. A fundamental error is for the leader to believe she should know everything, as others often believe! Her knowledge, however, must be sound and respected and she must be able to impart it to others. This knowledge is the foundation on which her confidence is built.

The leader must be true to herself; only then can she allow others to be themselves. One can assume a style of leadership but it is important to feel comfortable with it; an act will be recognised and respect lost. A knowledge of the different leadership styles is helpful as a model and the most useful is that which allows the team to use its initiative; this promotes staff motivation and growth. One should aim for the confidence to let people make mistakes (including the leader). A healthy mix of leadership styles may be predominantly democratic, laissez-faire from time to time and autocratic in certain situations when decisions have to be made. Staff need to feel safe by knowing who is in charge and under what style of leadership they are working; it must not change according to the mood of the leader.

The leader needs to know how to motivate the team when it is flagging, as it inevitably will. Motivation may be enhanced by praise and feedback (realistic and specific appraisal and fair and constructive criticism), and by giving time to people. Time spent with someone can say 'I value you and your contribution.' People need to feel valued before they can start to trust themselves and each other. It is important for the leader to feel secure in the organisation and have the confidence to recognise the skills, contributions and worth of each individual without feeling threatened herself. The leader needs also to encourage the team members to value each other; this corporate responsibility may be nurtured by example. Motivation may be enhanced by enthusiasm which, like disinterest, is contagious. However, it may be appropriate at times to accept that motivation is low and the team is at a low ebb.

The leader needs to allow for peaks and troughs in the life of a team. These do not indicate there is anything amiss with the leadership; they are a natural occurrence, particularly heightened when dying and death are an everyday event. One has to accept when the emotions of a team run high or low and encourage the team to have ordinary time together. A cup of tea or glass of sherry all round go a long way towards restoring a feeling of camaraderie. If the leader sets time aside for this to occur it gives the team a sense of value as human beings and permission is given for them to relax. The leader needs to create gaps in the timetable for sharing – sharing information, knowledge, problems and ideas. It is not the quantity of time available for communication that is important but the quality of that time.

The team leader needs to be aware of what the team wants and how it wants to function, and should allow time for discussion of these matters. She is also responsible for people knowing what is expected of them and the boundaries of their roles (a framework within which to work) and for ensuring that people are given the authority to act within these boundaries. Individuals within the team need structure and identity as much as the team itself.

The leader needs to exercise resource management and, as Vaughan and Pillmoor (1989) suggest, the leader is concerned with differentiating between the content of different work roles and then matching these with the team members available, according to their capacity for work.

The exercise of role definition by both leader and team member may help to ensure cooperation and understanding when allocating work within the team.

The leader is the person who 'worries' about the whole thing – who sees objectively what is happening within the team dynamics and who takes responsibility. A problem rarely goes away or resolves itself – if it is left in the hope that with time it will simply disappear, what happens in reality is that it grows and develops off-shoots. If (sometimes) painful pruning is not done early, the problem can proliferate and the end result is confusion and chaos: the staff feeling insecure and perhaps resentful and the leader feeling overwhelmingly helpless and a failure. This is particularly true of the 'team-splitter' and the 'difficult family'. It does not mean the leader has to have all the answers but her concern is to give the team confidence that it will not be abandoned to struggle with the problem alone – the leader will confront, listen and act appropriately. The leader needs to deal with disruption and not let it become acceptable.

Some Leader Coping Mechanisms

Leadership is a lonely position. For the leader to survive, remain effective and enjoy the role, looking after oneself is of prime importance. This means making space for oneself and being prepared to say no without feeling guilty. To be available, sensibly, means that everyone knows when one is not available. Effective leadership incorporates shrewd time management and this includes delegating responsibility and leaving work promptly. Staying late can soon become a way of life and should be avoided; it is not a good example to staff and can imply that they are not trusted to continue the work. In contrast, trusting staff may be beneficial to the leader, increasing staff development and competence. Most people respond to trust and the good relationship between the leader and staff engendered by this will be of mutual support.

The leader does not have to be infallible. Sharing with the team that one does not know, and admitting mistakes, such as ignoring a cue from a patient because of tiredness, may be endearing and even encouraging. Providing this is not a regular occurrence nor an indication of general incompetence it suggests that it is acceptable under this leader not to be perfect. The leader may also relax and not feel on show or on the defensive.

The leader's immediate manager plays a vital role in supporting the leader, by work appraisal and recognition of the leader's contribution and needs. It is important to allocate time on a regular basis for sharing ideas and updating each other. Furthermore, an hour a week spent with peers may prove invaluable as these are the only people who understand the stresses and frustrations as well as the rewards of the job. This time can be used to off-load onto colleagues and to learn from each other. By allowing this time within the working week the establishment is recognising the value and importance of its leaders.

The art of delegation may be the key to survival. The leader should not be hesitant to use the resources of the team. If the leader does everything herself people will let her because they think that is what she wants to do. Not only does this exhaust the leader but it inhibits the development of team members. And if delegation is the key to survival surely a sense of humour is the master-key.

Conclusions

There are no rules for team building. The dynamic nature of a team and the humanity of its members means that a team does indeed have to be built; and as the word implies this requires sustained effort. However, in order to address expertly the broad spectrum of issues and problems in palliative care (physical, emotional, social and spiritual) there is a need to provide care through an ID team. The product of a good working team is more than the sum of the individual members and this helps to create an optimal therapeutic environment.

References and further reading

BLANCHARD, K., AND JOHNSON, S. (1982) *The One Minute Manager*. William Collins Sons & Co. Ltd., Glasgow.

MANNING, M., (1984) *The Hospice Alternative, Living With Dying*. pp. 46–82. Souvenir Press Ltd., London.

VAUGHAN, B., AND PILLMOOR, M. (Eds.) (1989) *Managing Nursing Work*. pp. 29–44 Scutari Press, London.

ZIMMERMAN, J. M., (1981) *Hospice. Complete Care For The Terminally Ill*. pp. 97–125 Urban & Schwarzenberg Inc., USA.

Acknowledgements

The Nuffield Ward Interdisciplinary Team and in particular Jayne Sutcliffe for her invaluable contribution.

3

Tackling Total Pain

Mary Baines

Pain is a universal and unpleasant human experience. Its exact definition is far from easy, the most useful and simple being 'Pain is what the patient says hurts' (IASP Subcommittee 1980)

The easy assumption that the severity of pain is proportional to the extent of injury runs counter to both personal experience and clinical practice. A small boy may sustain a fracture while playing football and barely mention it. Similar degrees of arthritis appear to cripple one patient but, in another, be compatible with active life. Such common situations emphasise the fact that pain is subjective and is related both to tissue damage and to emotional factors. Pain is a somatopsychic experience.

If psychological factors modify the acute pain of trauma or the chronic but 'benign' pain of arthritis, it is to be expected that they will play an even greater rôle in the pain caused by advanced cancer. It was to emphasise this complexity of pain in the cancer patients with whom she worked that Saunders, in the later 1960s, first coined the phrase 'Total Pain' (Saunders 1967). She described this as having physical, emotional, social and spiritual components and she suggested that, unless each of these was tackled, pain relief was unlikely.

TOTAL PAIN

Physical
Emotional
Social
Spiritual

Fig 3.1

The term 'Total Pain' was to become central to the developing Hospice Movement. It became part of the foundation for the unique multiprofessional approach to the dying patient and his family which has become the hallmark of Palliative Medicine.

'Total Pain' is sometimes used to describe different aspects of *suffering* in the terminally ill. However, in this chapter the term 'Total Pain' will have its original and more restricted meaning, an approach to the patient who says 'It hurts'.

Total Pain – Physical Causes

The World Health Organisation estimates that 70% of patients with advanced cancer will suffer pain (W.H.O. 1986). Not all this pain is due to advancing malignant disease, it can be caused by debility, cancer treatment or 'benign' conditions such as arthritis or constipation.

Even when pain is caused directly by extending cancer it is important to make a diagnosis which should include the site involved and the pathological process. This diagnosis is the key to appropriate treatment. Some common causes of cancer pain are as follows:

- Bone pain from metastases.
- Tumour infiltration, compression or destruction of nerves.

- Visceral pain.
- Soft tissue infiltration,
- Intestinal colic.
- Lymphoedema.
- Raised intracranial pressure.

Total Pain – Emotional and Social Factors

It is probably quite rare for pain to be caused purely by non-physical factors. However, emotional and social problems frequently exacerbate pain and, indeed, a vicious cycle develops in which physical pain leads to anxiety or depression and they, in turn, lower the threshold for pain.

Poor communication between patient, family and staff is often the key to the problem. Most doctors and nurses find it is hard to talk with patients about their progressive illness and impending death. Families are often reluctant to discuss painful issues and prefer to keep their conversation to cheerful trivia. This conspiracy of silence leaves the patient feeling isolated or abandoned, trapped with his personal fears.

Such fears include how the disease will progress, and especially if it will lead to pain, incontinence or confusion. Then there may be major anxieties about the future of the family, particularly if there are dependent children, aged relatives or those with physical or mental illness. Worries over financial problems or unsuitable housing can also add to the patient's anxiety and so worsen his pain. Also the frustrations and boredom of prolonged dependency tend to make people focus on their bodily functions and their pain.

Total Pain – Spiritual Factors

Faced with serious illness or impending death many patients will begin to think more deeply about their life and its meaning. Some will have a profound sense of guilt and

failure about the past, things left undone or failed relationships. Others feel deeply the meaninglessness of life, that
there is no point or purpose in it. Some patients, especially
the old, long for death but feel guilty in so doing. A few are
troubled by the fear of what happens after death. The
religious patient – of any faith – or the convinced atheist,
may develop painful doubts as they face their terminal
illness. All these spiritual factors can cause anxiety and
insomnia, and so exacerbate pain.

Tackling Total Pain

This chapter is not a theoretical treatise on Total Pain but is
intended as a practical guide, outlining a plan of treatment
for the individual patient who complains of severe pain.

The first consultation should, if possible, take place with
one or more close family members present. This will enable
them to give their view of the situation, especially valuable
if the patient minimises his symptoms or is forgetful or
muddled. Their presence enables the doctor and nurse to
observe family interactions which may provide a clue to
some of the problems presented later.

After the routine clinical history a detailed description of
the pain is required. This should include site(s), severity,
duration, aggravating and relieving factors, response to
previous treatment and a verbatim description such as,
'like a red-hot poker' or 'painful pins and needles'. If
possible, a Body Chart, as described by Twycross (1984)
should be filled in by the doctor or nurse and patient
together.

Other symptoms are common and may exacerbate pain.
Details must be noted about appetite, vomiting, cough or
dyspnoea, weakness, bowel and bladder function, sleep
and mobility.

It is essential, but less easy, to enquire about the patient's
insight and mental state. Most doctors and nurses will
acquire phrases which seem appropriate for them, such as
'Did they talk to you much about the illness?', 'How did

you feel after all that?', 'What do you think has helped you cope with it all?' At this first consultation it is ideal to see the family alone, and also the patient alone, so that secrets in the family (usually concerned with diagnosis and prognosis) can be gently explored. The necessary physical examination should cover any signs relevant to the pain described, particularly any neurological deficit or local tenderness.

Such a comprehensive first consultation cannot easily be hurried, it may well take an hour or more. But it is time well spent, patients and families greatly value the opportunity to talk about their situation and this, in itself, is often therapeutic.

At the conclusion of such an interview, it is essential to list the problems presented and an approach to their management. This focuses thought, is invaluable for other members of the multiprofessional team, and for medical and nursing staff who may take over the care of the patient at a later date. Such a problem list may include distressing symptoms, lack of insight, anxiety or depression, family tensions, financial worries and perhaps a feeling of guilt or unworthiness. An example is as follows:

Mrs M.E. (45). Carcinoma of right breast with multiple bony metastases.

Problem	Management
Lumbosacral pain due to spinal metastases.	1. Nonsteroidal anti-inflammatory drug.
	2. Continue regular oral morphine. (may need dose increase)
	3. Contact R.T. Dept. re further R.T.
Constipation	Lactulose and Senna
Weakness	Encouragement Physiotherapy.

Problem	Management
Anxiety about the future. Poor communication with husband.	Meet husband, encourage them to be more open.
Boredom	Find out her interests. Involve Occupational Therapist.
Financial worries	Investigate possible grants.
Spiritual distress. Asking 'Why me?'	Time to listen. She would like to meet Chaplain.

In many situations such a list of problems can be made jointly by the doctor and nurse. It should then be shared with other members of the multiprofessional team and their views sought about the proposed management.

At this early stage it is rarely possible to estimate the extent to which emotional, social and spiritual factors contribute to the patient's pain. So the team must seek to advance on all fronts, tackling all the problems individually, while fully recognising that they interact and exacerbate each other.

Results of Treatment

Fortunately, the great majority of cancer patients have their pain relieved easily using simple drug regimens. After attending a week's workshop, Takeda returned to Japan to test WHO guidelines on the relief of cancer pain. (WHO 1986). He found that 87% of his patients became free of pain with drug treatment alone (Takeda 1986). Of course, this high success rate was with unselected patients, whereas hospices give preference to those with intractable symptoms. But these figures, and those from many hospices, show that the informed use of analgesics and adjuvant drugs, combined with the interest and enthusiasm of the staff will lead to good pain control in over 90% of patients.

Intractable Pain

Between 5% and 10% of cancer patients fail to obtain full pain relief. In some cases this may be due to poor compliance or a short time under treatment and others have severe but episodic pain. However, there remain a few who complain of severe, persistent pain which is partly or totally unresponsive to treatment. These are the patients whose predicament can overwhelm the multiprofessional team and who are not easily forgotten. They usually have a difficult physical pain, such as deafferentation, plus emotional, family and spiritual problems.

Effect on Team

The patient with uncontrolled 'Total Pain' generates a great deal of anger. He and his family may be angry with hospice staff, 'We came here because you said you could control pain'. The nurses will probably be angry with the doctors, feeling that they should do more. The chaplain and social worker feel frustrated – the patient says he cannot think about spiritual (or family) problems as he is in too much pain.

Occasionally, staff, especially new team members, feel that the patient is 'putting it on'. He may complain of pain while looking perfectly comfortable. He may ask for an injection but be asleep when the nurse arrives with it a few minutes later. In this situation the definition of pain needs to be emphasised. 'Pain is what the patient says hurts'. Cases of malingering (saying you're in pain when you're not) are virtually non existent. The pain caused (or exacerbated) by emotional factors is real pain and hurts. But its management may be different.

The Team Meets

In order to tackle the problem presented by the patient with uncontrolled pain it is essential for the team to meet regularly. This is relatively easy for the impatient; the ward doctors, nurses, social worker and chaplain will probably attend a weekly meeting at which the 'difficult patient' can be presented and discussed.

The patient at home will be under the primary health care team. General Practitioners and District Nurses may well feel frustrated and isolated in caring for patients with intractable pain and they will probably welcome meeting with some of the hospice staff who are also involved.

Such a team meeting will have two distinct purposes, sharing and planning, and it is most important for the leader to see that these two essentials are covered.

Just as patients are helped when they express feelings of anger or sadness, so are the staff supported when they can freely voice how they feel. 'He's never satisfied and always complaining', 'She doesn't respond to any treatment I've tried', 'I feel so angry at the way he treats his wife'. When such feelings are shared and perhaps understood, it is possible to go on, as a team, to plan the future strategy of care.

In the sections which follow, the contribution to the patient with severe uncontrolled pain of the nurse, doctor, social worker and chaplain, will be separately discussed. But, of course, these treatments are offered together, and the work of the team members will overlap. It is totally appropriate for the social worker to affirm the importance of regular analgesia, the nurse to teach simple quadriceps exercises and the doctor to pray with the patient who requests it.

In the cancer patient with really intractable pain it is rare for a single drug change, or family meeting, or talk with the Chaplain, to give relief. Much more often there is a gradual and partial response and it is quite impossible to determine which components of the multiprofessional team approach have proved effective.

The Nurse's Rôle

The patient and his family will see more of the nurse than any other member of the team. This is patently true for the inpatient but it is also true for the patient at home, for the great majority of those with advanced cancer who are having severe pain will be visited regularly by District Nurses. This close and continuing contact gives the nurse a unique opportunity to observe the patient in pain, and these observations are crucial for pain diagnosis and treatment. She will notice what causes exacerbations; walking, eating, or a visit from the family. The patient who gets relief of pain a few minutes after taking a tablet is suffering from anxiety rather than purely physical pain.

Some patients seem to use their pain to gain sympathy from an unsupportive family or attention from a busy nurse. It is more acceptable to say: 'Can I have something for my pain?' than 'I'm feeling low, please come and talk'. The observant Ward Sister will understand that these pains are really cries for help and she will try to arrange for nurses to visit regularly when the patient is not complaining.

It is the task of the Ward Sister to coordinate the multiprofessional team. They may suspect that a patient's pain is increased by her unwillingness to face her situation – but three staff members trying to have a meaningful discussion on the same day will be doomed to failure. The nurse, with her close contact with the patient and family, will often sense the appropriate time to raise these difficult issues.

The Doctor's Rôle

When pain fails to respond to conventional treatment, it is essential to have a complete re-evaluation of its physical cause. The pain may have been thought to be due to proven bone metastases, but a lack of response to radiotherapy and antiinflammatory drugs plus morphine should make the doctor rethink the diagnosis. A careful neurological examination and perhaps further investigations could lead to a diagnosis of deafferentation pain which requires a different therapeutic approach.

In Hospice practice, many of the 5%–10% with intractable pain do have evidence of nerve destruction (deafferentation). Records from a major Australian Pain Clinic show that about 30% of cancer patients who attend have deafferentation pain (Cousins M. J. 'Personal Communication 1989').

Having reviewed the diagnosis of the pain, new treatment options become apparent. Different adjuvant analgesic drugs can be used, for example, the tricyclic antidepressants are helpful for the constant aching pain caused by nerve destruction, while carbamazepine is better for shooting pain. (Tasker 1987)

Sometimes a different drug delivery system for morphine can be employed, the most valuable being by the epidural route. This is best used if the pain originally responded to oral morphine but the required dose now causes intolerable side effects (Cherry and Gourlay 1987). Other drugs which can be given epidurally are steroids and local anaesthetics.

The majority of patients with intractable pain respond, perhaps only partially, to these different therapeutic approaches combined with attention to emotional, social and spiritual distress. However, there remain just a few who get no better, despite all endeavours. The temptation for the doctor is continually to try new methods, to 'keep up hope'. But perhaps there is a place to admit failure, to accept – with the patient – that some degree of remaining pain seems unavoidable, and to reassure of continuing treatment and care.

The Social Worker's Rôle

The Social Worker has the enormous advantage of not being held responsible for pain control. As a member of the team, and being aware of the situation, he or she can open up a discussion with the patient and perhaps his family as well. 'It must be awful to have such a bad pain we can't do anything about'.

This will, almost inevitably, lead to a conversation in which anger and despair and fear are expressed. Anger at the previous treatment – or lack of it. Anger at false expectations raised – 'They said that the operation would help, but I've been much worse since then'. Anger at the 'incompetent' Hospice staff who 'can't get the drugs right'. Despair – 'Coming to the Hospice was my last hope, but I know now that I'll never be any better'. And fear – 'I am sure that the pain will get worse and worse and I'll die in agony – like my father'.

Having listened to the fears and anger caused by persistent pain, the Social Worker will be in a position to seek for emotional and social factors which could contribute to it. The question 'What do you think you'd be hurting about if you hadn't got this pain?' may bring up the patient's sadness at not going home, her worries about a sick husband or estranged children or financial need. There are rarely any easy or complete solutions to these problems, but the act of sharing with staff and family often relieves the anxiety which increases pain. Sometimes quite simple practical steps can be suggested. Making a will or specifying gifts for family or friends can give considerable satisfaction. Parents can be encouraged to make scrapbooks for their young children, reassuring them of their love and leaving memories of good times spent together. Patients often worry that their elderly relatives are neglecting themselves, being too occupied with care at home or hospital visiting. The offer of a Home Help, or transport, or financial support can relieve a great deal of unnecessary anxiety.

The Chaplain's Rôle

The Chaplain will be aware, perhaps more than others in the team, of the part which pain may play in the patient's life. Sometimes the pain is clung to as a means of getting sympathy or to prevent people from seeing the real person underneath.

Spiritual conflict, like anxiety, can increase pain. Perhaps the most common manifestations are a feeling of guilt about the past and a sense of the meaninglessness of life. Some people develop doubts about their previously strongly held beliefs and many feel that life is unjust or that they are being unfairly punished. Relatives often say – 'He's always led such a good life, he doesn't deserve this.' These feelings may be expressed to any sympathetic member of the caring team and all need to be sensitive to spiritual issues, able to listen, to offer help themselves or to seek skilled advice. Staff need to be aware of the relevant beliefs and practices of people of different faiths so that appropriate spiritual and practical help can be offered to these patients and their families.

Many Christian patients welcome the Chaplain's offer to pray with them. At this stage few are looking for physical healing so prayer is made for relief of pain or other distressing symptoms. And, as much of the distress of the dying is due to parting from the family, many patients appreciate the opportunity to pray with the Chaplain for those who will be left, entrusting them into God's care and keeping.

Support of Staff

Some staff have unrealistic expectations of what can be achieved. They seem to expect that all dying patients can be made painfree, without other physical distress, cheerful, accepting, at peace with their families and with God. It is the task of members of the multiprofessional team gently to remind each other that this is not often possible. The wise person can say: 'You're doing all right', or 'It's not perfect, but good enough'. For although the skills of nurse, doctor, social worker and chaplain are needed, and indeed, must continually be improved, the dying patient most needs them as people – those who will stay with him, in spite of his pain, and accompany him and his family to the end.

References

CHERRY D. A., and GOURLAY G. K. (1987). The Spinal Administration of Opioids in the treatment of Acute and Chronic Pain. *Palliative Medicine*. **1**: 89–106.

I.A.S.P. Subcommittee on Taxonomy (1980). Pain Terms: a list with definitions and notes on usage Pain. **8**: 249–252.

SAUNDERS C. M. (1967). The Management of terminal illness, *Hospital Medicine Publications*. London.

TAKEDA F. (1986). Results of Field Testing in Japan of the W.H.O. Draft Interim Guidelines on relief of Cancer Pain. *The Pain Clinic*. **1**, 83.

TASKER R. R. (1987). The Problem of Deafferentation Pain in the Management of the patient with Cancer. *Journal of Palliative care*. **2**: 2, p. 8–12.

TWYCROSS R. G. (1984). Relief of Pain. In the *Management of Terminal Malignant disease*. (ed C. Saunders) p. 64. Edward Arnold, London.

World Health Organisation (1986). *Cancer Pain Relief*, WHO Geneva.

PART II

Challenges to the Whole Team

4

Motor Neurone Disease

Betty O'Gorman and Tony O'Brien

Motor neurone disease is a disease of unknown aetiology characterised by progressive degeneration of the upper motor neurone tracts, the anterior horn cells of the spinal cord and the cranial nerve nuclei in the pons and medulla. The clinical presentation is often characteristic and the diagnosis must always be suspected when there is a combination of upper and lower motor neurone signs with no sensory loss. Three forms of the disease are described, reflecting the anatomical area which bears the brunt of the disease.

1. Progressive muscular atrophy. In this form, which affects primarily the anterior horn cells of the spinal cord and lower cranial nerve nuclei, the patient presents with asymmetrical weakness and wasting of the muscles of the hands, shoulder girdle and lower limbs. There may be an associated bulbar palsy with dysarthria and dysphagia. Examination confirms the weakness, wasting and fasiculation in the limbs.
2. Amytrophic lateral sclerosis. In this form the clinical picture is dominated by disturbance of upper motor neurone function. Patients present with stiffness in the legs

and a spastic paraparesis develops. Superimposed on this picture there may be signs of lower motor neurone involvement as shown by wasting and fasiculation.

3. Chronic progressive bulbar palsy. This form of motor neurone disease begins with involvement of the lower brain stem. There is progressive difficulty in swallowing, chewing and coughing, articulation and voice production. Patients lose weight rapidly and this form carries a poor prognosis.

Progressive muscular atrophy, amytrophic lateral sclerosis and progressive bulbar palsy are not distinct entities and in practice there is considerable overlap in the clinical presentation.

Sphincter control is preserved in motor neurone disease. While traditionally it was considered that intellectual function was not impaired, a proportion of these patients develop a dementing illness in the later stages.

Overall annual incidence rates for motor neurone disease are 1–1.5 per 100 000 population with a prevalence of 5 per 100 000. There is a consistent male excess of 1.5–1 and symptoms usually develop between 50–70 years. The mean survival is 3 years (6 months – 30 years).

Patients are referred for hospice care at varying stages throughout the disease. The aim of the team caring for patients with Motor Neurone Disease is to maximise each individual's potential and independence.

After the initial referral the GP will be contacted for permission to visit. Before the patient is seen the interdisciplinary team consisting of a doctor, home care nurse, social worker, physiotherapist and occupational therapist discuss which member of the team would be most appropriate to make the initial assessment. This is usually the home care nurse and physiotherapist. They will visit the patient and chief carers in the home setting, by appointment, at a time of day when the patient is least tired.

The assessment will be physical, emotional and social – not only of the patient but including the carers. The patient and carers need to be given time to describe the course the disease has taken to date. How is it now? How fast are things changing? What understanding have they of the disease? What are the specific problems? Who else in the community is involved and what is planned by them?

It is important at this visit to be prepared to spend time listening and empathising with their problems in order to be able to give practical help and information. It may also be appropriate to advise on drug management, the handling of the patient, ie lifting, transfers and support when walking, the consistency and type of food and drink, and bowel and bladder management.

It will become apparent what aids to daily living (ADL) will be helpful for the patient and carers. If possible these must be provided immediately or within a few days. The family needs to be left with a written plan of the services and agencies involved and how each will help.

The outcome of the visit needs to be reported back to the whole team. Soon after, if necessary, any other team members should be activated to visit and become involved with the patient.

All the community services and agencies involved will be invited to attend a meeting to plan the whole care of the patient and family. It is necessary to identify a key person from any of the disciplines involved, who has a full knowledge of all the areas where help may be obtained.

During the course of the illness it may be necessary to offer a respite admission for social and physical reasons eg family relief, symptom control, physical reassessment of the situation and alterations to the home. Or it may be that an admission is needed for terminal or continuing care. To relieve the anxiety of an admission the home care and in patient teams will liaise, with the physiotherapist acting as the co-ordinator having seen the patient both at home and then on admission. The patient will be cared for by a primary nursing team and will have daily physiotherapy.

The occupational therapist will assess and advise on new ways of doing everyday tasks with recommendations for alterations to the home environment where necessary.

The emphasis will be on what the patient can do at each stage of the disease and not on what they cannot do.

The social work department and chaplaincy will have become involved and it may also be necessary to liaise with or involve a speech therapist. Each patient requires a plan of care which is regularly reviewed. It should be structured, but not so rigid as to exclude informality and change and to take into consideration the patient's hopes, expectations and needs. He himself will be involved in this planning. Often management problems become apparent at the outset of in-patient care or sometimes at a later stage.

Ted Holden, who was an in-patient at St Christopher's Hospice, wrote 'An established routine, not rigid but encompassing the daily needs, is important. This would eliminate the irritation of having to repeat the struggle to be understood for simple predictable and constantly recurring things. Rapid staff changes are a real problem. It is helpful if they can be filtered in gradually with assistance as far as possible. That way mutual confidence is more quickly established. It is common for new people to be so tense that they become incapable of normal comprehension.' It is often difficult for the patient to express his frustrations. Ted Holden wrote 'Obviously and naturally my wife's visits have the greatest impact, but our very closeness means that we can more easily hurt each other and so we do have our problems, but we keep trying and considering the strains and tensions we manage pretty well. I believe that the main problem is simply to expect too much. One spends hours in eager anticipation which creates an oversensitive reaction to anything which falls short of expectation. The disappointment leads to poor communication and misunderstanding and as one realises that the mood is set and one is fully aware of the fundamental stupidity of it all, frustration, anger and remorse ensure that there is little prospect of recovery. What is sad is that you can do nothing until the next meeting which can be a long, long time.'

It needs the skill of the inter-disciplinary team to attempt to stay alongside such feelings. New members of the team (from any discipline) need emotional support and practical help from their more experienced colleagues.

Care of the patient may become difficult because natural preferences occur for different team members and their way of working. With continuing losses it is understandable that the patient may feel insecure, angry and become demanding in his behaviour. These problems have the potential of splitting the team. It could become necessary to address these problems with team members and the patient, to define boundaries.

As the disease progresses meetings with key team members, the patient and family will be arranged to address the changes and anxieties associated with the distress of deterioration. The family as a unit needs to remain intact. The value of their input as members of the caring team should never be underestimated. Partners need the space to be allowed to continue as a couple.

Hopefully total care of the patient and family will have evolved during the time the inter-disciplinary team has been caring for the patient, whether at home or as an in-patient. This continues through to death and to the bereavement care of the family.

To work in a team looking after a person with Motor Neurone Disease is often frustrating and exhausting. But to share with someone suffering from such a devastating disease is to see enormous courage.

Team members often become very fond of their patients and need to care for each other in their bereavement. Frequently many of them will want to attend the funeral.

Reference

TED HOLDEN. 'Patiently Speaking', *Nursing Times*, June 1980.

5

Twenty-four hours before and after death

Tony O'Brien and Barbara Monroe

The proper management of dying patients, together with the care of their family and friends, requires the skill of different professional groups. The patient is not just an individual with cancer who is dying, but a member of a family whose reactions interlock with his. The family is the unit of care and the way in which we handle the illness and death of their loved one will have an important influence on both their bereavement and their capacity to cope with future crises.

It is also important that staff who are caring for dying patients feel that they are doing a valuable and worthwhile job. This will only be achieved if they believe that the patients and families entrusted to their care receive appropriate medical, social and emotional support. However death is not always 'neat and tidy' and sometimes, despite our best efforts, patients are not as settled and as peaceful as we might like or expect. Occasionally death can be sudden and very distressing as when it happens in association with a major haemorrhage. In these instances, we rely on the support of each other so that no one person is overwhelmed with responsibility.

Medical Support

Most patients do not die suddenly of malignant disease. Normally there is a gradual deterioration during which patients spend increasing periods of time asleep. As they slip into a coma, they will be unable to take anything by mouth and finally a point is reached when death is clearly imminent. The time scale involved from the onset of coma to death is very variable and may range from just a few hours to a couple of weeks; typically death occurs within 24–48 hours.

When it is clear that death is approaching, and patients can no longer tolerate anything by mouth, prescribing priorities must change. The drug chart should be reviewed and all but essential medication stopped. A list of commonly used groups of drugs which can be withdrawn in the last 24 hours of life appears in Table 5.1.

Table 5.1 Drugs to withdraw in the last 24 hours

Corticosteroids
Non Steroidal Anti-inflammatory drugs
Antibiotics
Insulin/Oral Hypoglycaemics
Anti-depressants
Bronchodilators
Anti-Hypertensives/Anti-Arrythmics
Diuretics
Laxatives
Iron/Vitamin supplements

In considering what constitutes **essential** medication, the following guidelines apply:

- Adequate analgesic medication should continue to be given regularly, **even** when the patient is comatose
- Oral Anti-Convulsants may be replaced by Diazepam Suppositories, 10 mg–20 mg 8 hourly

- Hyoscine Hydrobromide should be used at the earliest sign of noisy breathing, in order to prevent the so-called 'death-rattle'
- Psychotropics (Phenothiazine/Benzodiazepines) should be continued by the rectal or parenteral route as appropriate and the dose titrated against the response
- Drugs should be charted and ready to be given by the nurse **without** further consultation with the doctor, in the event of some catastrophe, e.g. haemorrhage, fit.

Opioids

It is essential that adequate analgesic medication is continued. In the vast majority of patients, this involves the use of opioids. Diamorphine, because of its solubility, is the opioid of choice for parenteral administration. The conversion ratio of oral morphine: parenteral diamorphine is 3:1.

The diamorphine may be given by 4 hourly injections or may be infused subcutaneously by using a syringe driver. The choice between 4 hourly injections and a continuous subcutaneous infusion will reflect the preferences of the unit. In general, if the prognosis is less than 24–48 hours, 4 hourly injections have the advantage of allowing greater flexibility in doses. However, if it appears that the patient may live for some days, then the syringe driver is the preferred means of delivering the medication.

The suppository route may be useful in some instances, especially if the patient is dying at home. Oxycodone 30 mg 8 hourly = Morphine p.o. 15 mg 4 hourly. The use of morphine or dextromoramide suppositories in this setting is limited by their relatively short duration of action; 4 hours and 3 hours respectively.

Phenothiazines

These drugs may be used for their sedative, anti-emetic and co-analgesic effects.

Chlorpromazine may be given by injection (12.5 mg-50

mg 4–8 hourly) or as a suppository (50 mg-100mg 4–8 hourly). It cannot be used in a syringe driver.

Methotrimerazine is a potent antiemetic and analgesic with sedative properties twice as potent as chlorpromazine. It may be given by injection (25 mg-100 mg 4–8 hourly) and it can be used in a syringe driver. However, its use in the syringe driver is sometimes limited by the development of local skin reactions at the infusion site.

Hyoscine
This is a particularly useful drug in the last 24 hours. It has a variety of effects including:

Reduced secretions from exocrine glands
Smooth muscle relaxant
Marked sedation (rarely paradoxical agitation)
Anti-emetic

The dose of Hyoscine Hydrobromide is 0.4 mg-0.6 mg 4 hourly by injection, or it can be used in the syringe driver to a maximum dose of 2.4 mg/24 hours.

Benzodiazepines
These drugs are commonly used for the following effects:

Sedation
Muscle relaxant
Anti-convulsant

Diazepam 10 mg–20 mg may be given rectally 8 hourly. If this is not an option, Midazolam 10 mg–40 mg may be infused subcutaneously over 24 hours in a syringe driver.

In an emergency, e.g. bleeding and fits, nursing staff must have available medication which they can use without consultation with a doctor. Diazepam Rectal Solutions (Stesolid Enema) is a very rapidly absorbed form of diazepam which can be given without delay. Thus, in emergencies, it has certain advantages over the more traditional prescriptions of Diamorphine/Chlorpromazine/ Hyoscine.

Social and Emotional Support

Care of a dying person should be undertaken in a simple, unhurried fashion and with the minimum of fuss. Staff should be aware of the importance of maintaining a sense of dignity and identity for the patient even when he is unconscious. Family members need integrating into the caring team to whatever extent they feel comfortable. They can easily feel excluded by our professionalism and may welcome a suggestion that they should participate in the practical nursing care of the patient by helping with washing, moistening lips and so on.

We need to discuss with each individual whether or not they wish to be present at the time of death. Many people have not witnessed a death and may appreciate information about what to expect, how symptoms will be controlled and what will happen immediately after death. Time spent explaining the shift from oral medications to parenteral medication or the changing pattern of breathing will help to allay anxieties. Families under stress may wonder if the regular injections are contributing to the patient's deterioration and will value an opportunity to explore this.

Many relatives, and indeed staff, are distressed when a patient is unable to take food or even water. Explanation that nourishment is no longer of benefit to the patient may help. The desire to offer food and water is a powerful natural instinct but in this instance must be balanced against the patient's need for comfort. Intravenous hydration can be distressing and in a dying patient a degree of dehydration can actually improve comfort, in part by reducing troublesome bronchial secretions. A dry mouth can be treated with local measures.

Even at this late stage, there may be important things which family members need to say to the patient. It is always worth enquiring and surprising how often the answer is 'Yes'. If so, we need to ensure privacy and explain that although the patient is unable to show any response, he may well be able to hear.

The professional team must remember that death is a profound emotional and sometimes physical shock for relatives, however much it has been anticipated. At the time of death families need privacy to absorb what has happened, to say good-bye and to express their emotions in their own way. This is an opportunity for the family to unite in giving and receiving comfort and staff need to be careful not to intrude.

After this initial period relatives may welcome a suggestion of prayer; the calming voices and shared concern of others will help to contain the shock and panic brought on by the death. Prayer is important for many families and can provide considerable comfort. The prayers may extend to include members of the team, the other patients and their relatives. At a more basic level, the simple act of making and serving tea can introduce the familiar into a very unfamiliar situation.

After the death the body should be treated with care and respect. Particular attention should be paid to practices required by religion or culture. Family members may wish to help with washing and dressing the body and, if so, should be encouraged to do so. Other patients and their relatives should be told promptly and sympathetically that the death has occurred. It can be a source of strength and comfort for them to see that death was peaceful, that the dead are treated with dignity and their family with understanding.

The Day After

The family should be invited back to visit the ward on the day following death. Whenever possible, they should meet with a nurse who has cared for their relative, particularly if that nurse was also present at the time of death. By asking to see the family together we are making a clear statement of our concern for them. We can suggest that children should be included, but if they are not, perhaps suggest suitable books to read with them and discuss their need to grieve.

The meeting offers both the team and the family another chance to say good-bye and thank you. Endings are important; the family are losing not only the patient but the ward and the staff to whom they may have become very close. The bereaved need our acknowledgement of their pain and sorrow. Even if we have not had time to get to know a family, we can still offer them time to talk.

We can try to prepare the family for some of the otherwise bewildering physical and emotional experiences of bereavement. They need reassurance that it is normal to experience strong and conflicting feelings; love and resentment, sadness and anger. They need to know that 'if only's' are inevitable and that hearing the voice of the dead person does not mean you are going mad. We can help grief by sharing a personal memory of the dead person and by expressing our own sadness. This often acts as a trigger to help the bereaved start the necessary but painful process of remembering.

The past is important. Families may need to rehearse the details of the illness and death before they can begin to say good-bye to it. If they were not present at the time of death it can be helpful for a nurse who witnessed it to describe clearly what happened. Relatives may need encouraging to ask questions and to hear our answers: 'Should I have let him come into the hospice sooner? Did that last injection cause his death?' People need to feel that they did what they could and it is important to validate their care of the patient and to remind them of their own strengths and achievements.

Another function of the meeting is to encourage acceptance of the reality of death. We can allow the family to read the death certificate for themselves. Using the past tense and words like 'dead' and 'cancer' helps to reinforce reality as does the process of collecting possessions. Relatives need clear and practical advice about such matters as how and where to register the death, finances and how to arrange the funeral. People under stress forget easily and information should be written down, most usefully in the form of a standard leaflet. Differences in grieving can create tensions within families, for example allowing someone to cry is not the same as implying that they ought to do so. We can help people to acknowledge these differences and to give one another permission to grieve in their own way and their own time.

Individuals also differ about whether or not they wish to view the body. There is no right or wrong option and individual choices should be respected. We should indicate early in the meeting that there will be an opportunity to view the body and describe where it is and how it will look so that people can make an informed decision. Relatives who wish to view may be accompanied by a member of staff who can encourage the family in verbal good-byes or a physical embrace, by themselves gently touching the body. Some people will simply want to spend some time sitting quietly with the body and there should be comfortable surroundings in which they can do so.

Finally, this after death meeting offers us the chance to assess people's risk in bereavement and if appropriate to refer them on to a bereavement service. We should remind ourselves, however, that the patient was not our property and neither is his family. Grief is a normal and inevitable human journey, not an illness. Most people will success-fully accomplish the tasks of grief with the help of their family, friends and local community.

6

'Intractable' Symptoms

Bridget Wood

Any symptom can become intractable. That is not just difficult to control, but unyielding to any treatment or intervention – something the patient is stuck with. In some cases the symptom presented is the inevitable consequence of advancing malignant disease. For instance weakness, the symptom most commonly complained of on admission to St. Christopher's Hospice. Steroids or physiotherapy may give temporary improvement, there is much that can be done to aid the patient's independence and improve his sense of wellbeing, but as the disease advances increasing weakness will accompany it. Faced with many other symptoms (generalised pruritis, hiccough, malignant sweats to name but a few) we work through the list of textbook remedies with little enthusiasm, knowing current medical expertise has limited success in alleviating them.

So how does an interdisciplinary team approach the management of intractable symptoms? As patients with terminal illness come to terms with their limited prognosis they are often helped by recognising it is possible to simultaneously hope for the best and prepare for the worst. Perhaps as the team approach the care of patients with difficult symptoms they can hold in tension continuing efforts to alleviate the symptom and taking steps to prevent an intractable symptom establishing itself as an intractable problem.

At the first meeting between a member of the team and the patient a careful assessment of each symptom and consideration of the likely cause for it is the starting point for establishing realistic expectations for what may be achieved in control of that individual's symptoms. A simple example would be a patient presenting with a typical history of subacute intestinal obstruction, perhaps from intra-abdominal carcinomatosis due to carcinoma of the ovary. With extensive intra-abdominal carcinomatosis surgical correction of obstruction is usually impossible. However, it is well established that with the use of anti-emetics, analgesics and antispasmodics, often delivered via a syringe driver, it is almost always possible to control nausea and abdominal pain caused by the obstruction. Vomiting is minimised, but if the patient's nausea is well controlled and she continues to eat and drink as she pleases (which is encouraged), it is usual for intermittent vomiting to continue. Normally the patient will experience only a short period of nausea or epigastric fullness before the vomit, vomiting will occur only once a day or less, and once the patient has vomited she rapidly feels better again. If this is explained to the patient in advance, the vomiting – which could be seen as an intractable symptom, is usually accepted by the patient as a mild nuisance, rarely is it complained of as a significant problem.

Often there will be a mismatch of expectations between the professionals, the patient and family. In the patient's mind the team may have been billed as 'the experts', raising hopes for improvement beyond the realms of possibility. A doctor visiting St. Christopher's said he had come to find out 'how you give all your patients a great sense of wellbeing . . .' Presumably he also transmitted this expectation of Hospice to his patients! Alternatively, the patient's past experience, perhaps involvement in the care of a relative with cancer many years ago, may have left them with very negative expectations. For example, it is still an astonishingly common misconception that all patients with cancer die in terrible pain.

Naturally, caring professionals, whilst trying to convey an honest and realistic view of what symptomatic improvement the patient may expect, are influenced by their own expectations – modified by individual experience. We protect ourselves from 'failing' in the eyes of ourselves and others. We are aware that we will lose the trust of patients and their families if we are over-confident and don't 'deliver the goods'. But equally wary of pessimism, knowing that the enthusiasm and confidence (or lack!) of the giver does transmit itself to the patient, and is an important influence on the efficacy of the treatment suggested.

One member of our team said 'by talking things through I find out if my goals are realistic.' Discussion within and across disciplines, and the possibility of 'second opinions' . . . critical re-appraisal by other members of the team, allows us to be sure we have covered all the options, and often to be affirmed in a difficult situation. Without this we can be left with niggling doubts . . . 'am I missing something?' With the benefit of colleagues to 'talk things through' it is certainly easier to define goals and to acknowledge our limitations, allowing us to approach the patient on a firm footing from which we can help them towards realistic expectations.

Surely one of the most crushing things ever said to a patient facing a terminal illness is 'we can do no more for you.' If an unpleasant symptom does prove to be truly intractable we have to find some way of 'staying with it', continuing to support the patient and family despite the persisting symptom (even allowing a patient to ventilate his feeling about a symptom may help its not being ignored). Often it will be possible without minimising the particular symptom to improve the general comfort and quality of life for the patient in other ways. Certainly we should avoid becoming so fixated by one difficult symptom that we neglect other symptoms and aspects of the patient's care.

For ourselves, natural feelings of failure in this situation may be helped by being able to honestly acknowledge and share our disappointment within the team. And the load is spread because the patient and family are cared for by more than one individual in the team. Whilst we are never complacent about 'intractable symptoms', nor should we dwell exclusively on negatives, it helps to recognise our successes and usefulness within the overall picture. When a member of our team reported back to us having spent several hours of the previous night at a particularly difficult home death and the whole team, knowing the patient and family, felt very low, another member was able to say 'imagine how it would have been if you hadn't been there.' Sometimes as we grit our teeth to 'stay with it' we need to allow ourselves to see this other perspective.

In our more frustrated moments it can help to remember that advances in symptom control are being made all the time. A recent example is the control of lymphoedema. The massage and bandaging techniques pioneered by Caroline Badger have been very successfully employed at least for temporary relief of this distressing and disfiguring symptom in several of our patients. A continued curiosity in new treatments and a willingness often to learn across disciplines as well as across specialities within medicine will ensure we continue chipping away at our pile of intractable symptoms.

At times the professional carer will face disappointment and anger from the patient stuck with his awful symptom and from his family who perhaps expected more improvement. Often the anger directed against the professional for his/her 'failure' is more truly anger over the presence of the symptom and underlying disease and all that that implies than anger actually engendered by any individual for failure in controlling a symptom, but it can feel very personal. Again a team who work well together are able to share 'the blame' and the stress of this situation. It may be of particular value to the family in such circumstances that more than one member of the team (and where appropriate two or more team members of different disciplines) has assessed the patient, this being an added reassurance to them that every avenue is being explored to help the individual.

Often in fact we are struck by the amazing generosity of patients and families, who do appreciate our 'sticking with it,' and view this as continued care and support rather than point out what we consider our continued failures! Often indeed we probably spend more time with patients whose symptoms are 'intractable' than those where symptom control proves straightforward. Whilst this is probably an overprotective compensation for our helplessness, we may unwittingly be providing the form of support they most value.

Finally, in a small proportion of cases where symptoms appear intractable it may be worth considering whether for some reason the patient needs the symptom. Is there a secondary gain, whether conscious or subconscious? A lonely or frightened patient who is unable to express this, or feels no-one will listen may 'demand' attention by persistently presenting a physical symptom. A patient who has adopted the 'sick role' within a family (and often been enforced in this by repeated hospitalisation and visits of health carers) may cherish the additional attention and affection received from the family, and fear losing this if they are shown to be capable of greater independence as we strive to control their symptoms and fulfil our hopes for them.

Occasionally a patient may use a physical symptom as a persistent focus to avoid looking at his cancer and its deeper implications at all. A man of forty-two with extensive pelvic tumour due to carcinoma of the rectum was troubled by diarrhoea from his colostomy. As he grew weaker he insisted that the loss of fluid from his colostomy was 'draining away' his strength. If this could be controlled, he argued, he would be fine again. He was aware that he had extensive cancer but certain that he could live with his cancer if only the diarrhoea was stopped. In fact he was still eating and drinking well and was not dehydrated, undoubtedly his rapidly progressing cancer was the cause of his weakness. This was a form of denial, he protected himself from the pain and anger that facing the truth would have caused. He died at home, having maintained this defence and without ever openly acknowledging he was dying.

7

The Team Splitter

Helene Channon

It is the purpose of this chapter to consider the problem posed to the multi-professional team by the 'team splitter,' a problem which may be produced by either a patient/ family member or a team member. Neither of them make us feel at all comfortable, both need attention if the team is not to be split.

Firstly then, the problem patient or family member. Who are these problem individuals and how is it they disrupt team life?

In discussion with my own team it was agreed that patients most likely to disrupt our group and effective work together were the longer term patients or those very dependent on our care. We agreed that differing expectations were a key factor as was poor inter-team communication and, ultimately, lack of trust both within and across the various disciplines.

An example might be a patient with motor neurone disease. Often their degree of paralysis means they are totally dependent on our care. Unless we communicate with the patient clearly about our working practice and agree a plan of care, to be regularly reviewed, differing expectations and aims will soon result and team conflict emerge.

At St. Christopher's, the system of team nursing means that a small team of four or five nurses will be responsible for the total care of a group of patients from admission through to discharge or death. In our experience, this has reduced the kind of conflict previously met with when any one of eighteen staff might care for any group of patients each day.

Agreeing a plan of care with the patient and, where appropriate, his/her family also, reduced the likelihood of conflict. Reducing the number of 'cooks' has proved a useful way of avoiding persistent change of approach to particular aspects of care, such as the dressing of pressure sores, or positioning the quadraplegic MND patient so that he may sit without discomfort.

The benefit to the multi-professional team is the improved insight and awareness of the smaller group of patients that each team caring for them will gain.

Both within and across the disciplines trust is a vital ingredient if the team is to survive and function as a team as opposed to a group of individuals. I would suggest that trust is established and nurtured by respect and open and honest communication. We need too to acknowledge the strengths of the team members from different disciplines and to work at thinking in terms of the whole team and the contribution that each individual has to make, when decisions are to be made. This is especially necessary when the demands made on us by a patient or family member threaten our team's stability. An example might be the family member who blames their relative's drowsiness and deterioration on the medication prescribed rather than see it in the context of their relative's deteriorating condition.

Conflict of ideas, aims and expectations needs to be thrashed out if a team is not to be split. The multidisciplinary team will have to be accustomed to being together and to communicating openly if this is to be done effectively. If I trust someone I am not afraid to disagree with them. The same must be the case when the potential team splitting situation is discussed. The best solution in our experience has been the calling together of the whole team, the airing of the problem and possible ways ahead being batted around. When the team has communicated adequately together, the patient and/or family member might then be involved. The same process will apply and a plan of action agreed.

In caring for longer term patients we have realised the need to meet as a team together with them and their family at regular intervals. These provide an opportunity for care to be reviewed, grievances on both sides to be aired and to set a pattern of communication. The same also applies in our care of shorter term patients. For both groups unshared truths and consequent different expectations might often be explored at such meetings.

Perhaps, however, of the two potential team splitters, the problem team member, from whichever discipline, is the more uncomfortable.

When considering who the team splitter from within the multidisciplinary team might be, we agreed that often they were people who had a poor concept of a team for a variety of reasons including a poor previous experience of such a team approach. This may be a person who needs to 'do their own thing,' and needs to be everything to each patient or to the patient they are currently caring for. They are often people who feel indispensible and may consequently also become over involved and are perhaps people who are looking to meet their own needs, none greater than the need to be needed. They are sometimes lazy individuals who take no responsibility for team life.

The effect on members of their own discipline and other disciplines may well be anger or frustration. Confusion often arises as what is communicated by this individual might be in conflict with the team opinion and what should be a team perspective becomes an individual perspective and possibly narrow or incomplete.

Dealing with a problem team member is not easy. (This may especially be the case if they are the only representative of their profession). Essentially the problem is a managerial one and as such, once it has been perceived as a team problem, the individual's manager should be approached and the situation explained. As the manager of the largest group within the multi-professional team I am of course also responsible for the initial handling of any nurse who is creating problems.

Confrontation should always be handled assertively, that is communication needs to be clear: problems need to be dealt with one at a time and without putting down the individual who has been found to be a problem.

It is totally appropriate for me as the nurse manager of the ward nursing team to share problems across the disciplines if I see the problem as one which will potentially split the team. There is no room within real multi-professional team work for an inappropriate protectiveness or defensiveness towards one's own profession. Again, open, honest communication across the whole group is necessary if the members are to trust each other and function fluently in the care of patients, families and one another.

A team which is unstable for whatever reason might be more likely to split, as its instability and therefore perhaps lack of identity gives licence to individuals to 'do their own thing.'

At St. Christopher's it is agreed that the ward sister manages the ward team. It is imperative for each profession and for the team as a whole that liaison is with an identifiable person. My role is to see that none are overlooked or undervalued. Each team, especially one that is unstable, needs to know the identity of its leader in order that its own identity in times of 'flux' might not be lost.

By way of summary I should like to close this chapter with a short example of the problems posed to a multidisciplinary team by the 'team splitter.'

Soon after becoming ward sister a staff nurse joined the ward team and in a short time caused a considerable amount of disruption. She was intelligent and considered 'dynamic' by her colleagues. It seemed however that her ability to work within a team had yet to be proved. She had strong ideas about the right way of going about things and would often over-rule decisions regarding nursing care and communicate these aggressively to members of her own discipline and persuasively to those of other disciplines. This initially gave rise to a certain amount of conflict between members of the different disciplines. She very quickly became attached to patients and would often stay late in order to speak with and meet their families. This created a tension amongst the nursing team and a certain amount of frustration across the professions as patients and families would assume that this was the norm.

Before confronting her and aside from praying for grace and wisdom to deal with the situation, I spoke with our ward consultant, social worker and physiotherapist. I discussed in brief the problems identified and the desire to see this individual settled and become a part of our ward team, so that what she had to give became the focus, and not anything less. We agreed that they would each come to me if they observed any of the behaviour highlighted as a problem.

I then saw the staff nurse and together we agreed and set behaviour targets, things she knew she was to aim at achieving in the ensuing months. Some of these targets would pose no problem, some would take more effort. We also agreed on a pattern of communication. I explained the philosophy of team nursing and asked her not to involve herself with any of the patients or families outside her designated group nor outside of her on duty time. In addition, I saw and worked with her regularly.

I communicated this programme to the senior team representatives of all the disciplines. By the time she left to take up a more senior position, this staff nurse, a potential team splitter, had become a much valued team member.

8

Stress and Frustration in Home Care

Barbara Saunders

We use these words in everyday language; it is therefore good to discover whether we really know the correct meanings.

- **Stress** is demand upon physical or mental energy.
- **Frustration** is to be discontented through inability to achieve one's desires.

A Friday evening at the end of a busy week seemed to be the best time to gather together our inter-disciplinary Home Care Team to 'brain storm' this subject. On this occasion there were seven nurses, two doctors, a social worker and secretary. Our occupational therapist was not available but she added a few ideas later.

Let me explain how and where we work just to put our frustrations and stresses into context. We are an advisory and supportive team working in outer London, visiting patients with cancer, and a few with motor neurone disease, who have been referred for home care by their General Practitioners or hospital Consultants (but only seen with GP permission).

- We visit in an approximate seven mile radius from the hospice and cover a population of about two million. Housing in this area is mixed, consisting of council flats, small houses, smart apartments, up to large detached houses. The patients and families likewise come in all shapes and sizes and from very poor to wealthy. Nevertheless, different though they all are, the patients are smitten with a life threatening illness and their loved ones are suffering with them.
- We have between 30–45 patients referred each month and have between 75–85 patients on our list at any one time. We run a 24 hour service, and have back-up beds available in the Hospice.
- We work with the primary health care team and do not take over the care of patients but offer advice and extra time to listen as families work out their problems.

It was interesting to note from our 'brain storming' list that there were more stresses than frustrations so we will look at the former first.

Lack of time was high on the list; it is hard to refuse to take on another patient whose need is great. We can never say the beds are full as an in-patient unit may say. Nevertheless we have had to learn to say 'no', else our service would be so diluted that it could become of no use, but the increasing waiting list at times is certainly stressful.

Being called out at night is stressful, particularly when, for example, the caller leaves a message from a phone box saying 'Come quickly, mother is very ill' and you could not phone back to get further details because the family did not have a telephone; it is midnight and you do not know the route but you do know it is in an area where people do not go by choice at night. On another occasion you give some advice over the phone because there is no need for you to visit; you return to bed and toss from side to side 'of course you should have gone', 'I've probably killed him with my advice', 'I'm just lazy'. The next night on call you go out, still wondering whether it is really necessary, after all the family do have a night sitter. On arrival you are greeted with total abuse, 'why did you take so long', 'she's dead' – 'go away'. What does the stress of a family member's anger do to you?

How do we anticipate patients' needs?

- Will she be able to continue taking her drugs by mouth, should I be asking her G.P. to prescribe injections, what happens if she can't take her 10.00 p.m. oral morphine? Will the G.P. think I'm over-reacting? Will the family think I am alarmist?
- Should I ask that son in France to return from his holiday?
- Do you think he could manage that journey to Eastbourne to say 'goodbye' to his mother in the Nursing Home?
- Should I get a night nurse tonight?
- Should I plan for him to be admitted tomorrow?
- How do I live with my mistakes? I persuaded him to be admitted for a couple of days to try to better control his pain and he's died, would he have lived for longer at home? His wife so wanted to keep him there.
- Why didn't I prescribe him anti-biotics, just once more?
- Why didn't I think of trying this drug or that treatment?
- Why didn't I listen?
- Why was I impatient?
- Why don't I like her?

Then there is the stress of patients never getting better – why do they all have to die?

Watching the grief of families is so stressful. The new wife of three weeks whose dying husband had been a childhood sweetheart, but they had gone their separate ways until six months ago – true happiness had only just been found, only to be cruelly snatched away. Sometimes a child will say innocently 'Is Mummy going to die?' What do you do with that pain?

How much does it hurt when your colleague shares that with you – how can you help her to bear it?

Your colleague's anguish that you try to share may not, of course, be from the patients. It may be his or her own family problems that can't be kept a secret any longer and come tumbling out. Or the trauma of that car crash on that wet road, just another stress at the end of a busy day.

Then we have different stresses, trying to maintain high standards all the time, after all we are told that we work in a place of excellence, you must not let the side down!

We have students out on visits, we enjoy sharing with them and they are keen to learn but it all takes time. Then we have the pressure of teaching and yet there are new patients to be clerked and which is most important? Patients, of course, so another evening is spent at home on preparation.

So to progress to our frustrations: they lie, for example, in asking a G.P. to prescribe but he won't be persuaded to give what we are sure will help. Or he declines to visit when we believe he should, or he will not even permit a visit from us, when referral has come from hospital and we think we could help.

Frustrations also come from interpersonal team conflict. We all have 'off days'; we cannot always be pleasant all the time, nor do we necessarily all like each other all of the time and some of the other stresses make these frustrations harder to bear.

Arriving late for meetings causes frustration, giving the group insufficient time and making others late for the next meeting.

Then there is the frustration of those who are willing to stay late at night and arrive before the others in the morning. How do the rest of the team feel – perhaps lazy or second class!

Having looked at some of the stresses and frustrations let us now look at the positive side of how these problems can be avoided or relieved. It needs to be remembered that a certain amount of stress is beneficial. It keeps us alert and striving for good care and for job satisfaction. Where there is no tensions, the person can become bored and disinterested.

Selection, by a small inter-disciplinary group, of the right team members is the start of stress prevention. Ideally, a team should consist of those who have not suffered recent losses or those who have come to terms with earlier losses.

Staff with good clinical and pharmacological skills, those who can think on their feet; Those with a good sense of humour and those who listen and communicate well. The right balance of team members is important, the extroverts and the thoughtful, the ideas people and those who are sensitive to the needs of others, to give but a few examples.

It is especially desirable for them to have outside interests, remembering that life doesn't begin and end at work, therein lurks trouble. Apart from the mental and physical health of the team member, other interests make a more interesting visitor for the patient.

Each member needs to be genuinely appreciated and each needs to be appraised regularly, to be encouraged and guided to build his self-confidence. Each needs to be made aware of colleagues' needs, to support one day and to be supported another. Even routine events such as the ritual coffee can be used as a team building time. (Spend some money on a good coffee maker and some attractive cups). There is something about serving coffee on a tray to others that is part of caring for each other, as long as the serving is shared. There is certain stress in always being the one who makes the coffee and washes the cups!

Celebrating together, remembering the birthdays (good cake makers in the team are essential). These are treats to enjoy. The right balance must be obtained in meeting together. Celebrating Christmas and having parties can be times for get togethers, and opportunities to show appreciation.

Team members also need to make time to have lunch breaks, they are opportunities for relaxation and socializing, they can so easily be missed.

All these aspects are important, but the greatest scheme for preventing stress is inter-disciplinary team working. Debating the needs of patients together, tossing around ideas until the best solution is reached. Encouraging, teaching, learning, listening, sharing with each other. Being able to laugh with each other, seeing the funny side of life; as well as the serious and the sad. Being open and honest with feelings, doubts and mistakes, reduces tension to both the individual and the team as a whole.

The gratitude of families, their lovely and often moving letters of thanks, are a great source of encouragement. At our Annual Memorial Service, families' appreciation is a great help in inspiring us to carry on. The knowledge that they are learning to live their lives again is also gratifying.

Continued training and the following of special interests and projects can prevent stress. Teaching in itself gives a very good balance to the work, somehow by teaching others by giving examples of experiences and of mistakes helps stress to be talked out and, hopefully, guides others away from similar pitfalls. This teaching by a cross section of the inter-disciplinary team and sometimes with members of the primary care team, can be very effective in demonstrating how a team works together.

It is important to consider finally whether stress and frustration can lead to exhaustion, perhaps common parlance would be 'burn out' or 'battle fatigue'. Of course, this can and does occur but can certainly be avoided, if as already discussed, proper preventative measures are taken, namely that team members are properly selected, educated, supported and encouraged. That they learn to share together as an inter-disciplinary team. That they acknowledge their limits and those of their colleagues. By taking this path there may be a few sparks but certainly not a bonfire.

9

The Difficult Family

Alison Virdee

Even the title of this chapter conjures up the negative feelings a team may have when faced with a family who overwhelm them. The reasons for these feelings emerging are varied and may be different for each team. The effect is that they feel unequal to the challenge of assisting that family in their need to make sense of their situation and cope with it. I would like to describe such a family and discuss the ways in which our team tackled the problems.

Firstly, we have found that clear, precise documentation of the family history in the medical and nursing notes enables any member of the team to have access to the facts of the situation. So I will draw a 'family tree' of the family I am going to describe.

Mrs. Amble was a 58 year old woman suffering from carcinoma of the lung. She was admitted to St. Christopher's Hospice with severe dyspnoea and was anxious on admission. Her religion was given as 'Church of England' but she was not a churchgoer. She was a strong and capable household manager for her extended family who were all still living at home or in the same street. She found it very hard to accept help from others and could not rest. Most of the communication in the family happened through her and she had mediated in all family disputes.

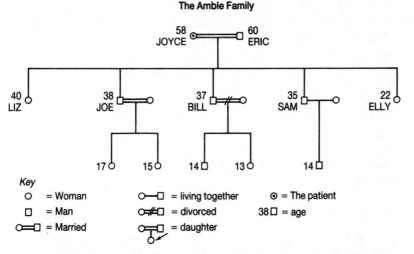

The Amble Family

Key

O = Woman   O—☐ = living together   ⊙ = The patient

☐ = Man   O≠☐ = divorced   38☐ = age

O═☐ = Married   ⟨daughter symbol⟩ = daughter

Mr. Amble was a quiet, indecisive man who had always deferred to his wife's judgement. He appeared isolated in this large family and was distressed when visiting.

Liz, the eldest daughter, was extremely close to her mother and still lived at home. She had been unable to come to terms with her mother's illness and seemed unrealistic about the present situation.

Elly, her youngest daughter, was disabled by cerebral palsy and was wheelchair bound. Her mother had cared for her all her life and fought all her battles with the Social Services. Elly had difficulties with physical care and benefits but felt unable to deal with these.

Bill, her middle son, had had an alcohol problem for a few years and was often drunk and abusive when visiting.

The grandchildren were half brought up by Mrs. Amble and were very upset by her illness. They were quite noisy and disruptive in the ward and seemed unsupervised.

Joe and Sam were close and supportive of the family, who visited in large groups at variable times of day. Mrs. Amble loved their visits but tended to do too much and became dyspnoeic when they were there. This frightened the family as they feared she would choke and die suddenly. On admission, a detailed family history was taken, along with medical details, by a doctor and a nurse. This was recorded as a 'family tree' in the medical and nursing notes and contact telephone numbers and addresses for family members were also taken.

After a couple of days of getting to know this family the team began to feel quite overwhelmed and confused about how to help them. It was decided by the ward sister to discuss the Amble family in the weekly multi-professional meeting. Below are some of the problems that were discussed at the meeting and what decisions were made.

Problem Discussed	Decision/Action
1. Sheer size of the family and number of people on the ward at all times of the day. 'They seem to be everywhere, all the time!' They all ask a lot of questions and take a lot of staff time.	Nursing staff to set rules about numbers of visitors and allocate another place for the family to go when not with Mrs. A. For all staff to accept that this is a large family and not to panic! Try to get to know who is who and feel less overwhelmed. Arrange a meeting with the whole family, social worker, nurse, doctor, so they can ask all their questions together.
2. Mrs. A's anxiety and dyspnoea which does not seem to respond to medical treatment, is worse when family visits and this frightens them, which makes her more anxious, etc. etc.	Physiotherapists to practice 'pacing herself' and relaxation exercises with cassette tapes. Visiting rules will help to calm the situation. Discuss dyspnoea and anxiety with the family in the arranged meeting to give them medical details. Chaplain to investigate any spiritual component to anxiety.

3. Communication is very poor in this family as Mrs. A. used to be the central figure.

Use arranged meeting to discuss this with family and try to get them to nominate a central figure for the staff to contact. Then they can pass on information to the rest of the family.

4. Elly's problems with benefits etc.

Social worker to contact her own district social worker and inform her of the changes in circumstances.

5. Bill's bad behaviour on the ward.

All staff to treat him the same way as the rest of the family Answer questions, etc but if he becomes threatening or abusive call the police to take him away. Warn the family that we would do this.

6. Mr. A. seems isolated in this family.

Whole team to make sure he does not get lost in the family. Social worker to spend some time with him alone to assess how he is coping.

7. Liz's unrealistic ideas about her mother's illness.

Make sure that diagnosis and prognosis are discussed in the arranged meeting. Nursing staff to check out afterwards if she was able to take it in. If not refer to social worker for further assessment.

8. Grandchildren seem unsupervised.

Nursing staff to tell family that all children must be accompanied when visiting. Discuss the different needs of children and teenagers in this situation. Set up a meeting for just grandchildren with social worker, nurse, doctor for them to ask questions and discuss worries.

So, as a team, we had discussed the fact that we should allow ourselves to be merely human and accept that this set of problems was too large and complex for us to 'fix' them all. Some problems had existed for many years and all we could do was limit the damage that occurred while the family were in our care. However, we could try to identify a few ways in which we were able to help. We could improve family communication; reduce tension and anxiety to alleviate Mrs. Amble's symptoms; anticipate bereavement problems in some members of the family. We were able to identify ways of helping that would give the family structured attention that they needed and reduce the feeling of chaos for staff in two meetings and by setting a few ground rules. This helped the whole team to feel calmer, less overwhelmed and more in control and we agreed to tackle only the problems we may be able to help with, and the Amble family did not feel quite so impossible any more.

The family accepted the new ground rules and spent most of their time, in large groups still, in the family lounge off the ward. They also nominated Joe as the central family member for communication. Mrs. Amble gradually became less anxious as she saw her family taking responsibility for themselves and coping. Her husband managed to communicate that he would like some time alone with his wife and this helped both of them to share their feelings. Liz and the rest of the family were able to clarify the details of Mrs. Amble's illness and prognosis and they were reassured that she would not die choking and that staff would control pain and discomfort when she became less well. Elly started to liaise more with her District Social Worker about her financial problems. Bill continued to arrive drunk on the ward and was occasionally abusive when visiting but staff felt confident in asking him to leave and he always left promptly.

Three weeks later Mrs. Amble had a series of episodes of haemoptysis and deteriorated quite quickly. She died 24 hours later, very peacefully with her husband and children sitting by the bedside. Bill did not feel able to cope with this and was informed of his mother's death by telephone.

When we looked back at the management of this family the team felt that overall the family's time on the ward had been more calm and positive than they could have hoped for. By improving family communication and structuring the attention they received, the Amble's were able to spend the last three weeks in the way they each needed but also in a way that was possible for the ward team.

10

Supporting Children Facing Bereavement

Barbara Monroe

Children facing the death of a parent or close relative arouse strong feelings in us all. They remind us of ourselves as children and of our own children or the children we hope for. Their vulnerability makes us acutely aware of the possibility of damage, of doing or saying the wrong thing. We want to protect children but in doing so we often exclude and isolate them. To protect a child from the truth is to leave him confused, unprotected from his fantasies and unsupported with his feelings. Many of us will have met adults whose ability to handle emotional crises has been profoundly damaged by a misunderstood or ignored childhood bereavement.

Terminal illness causes enormous changes within the family and children can sense when something so serious is happening. However, many parents, like professionals, know little about children's reactions to illness and death and decide to delay telling them 'until later, until they're old enough to understand'. It is precisely because children do not understand what death is all about that they need to talk about it. Ideally they need preparation before the death; a chance to ask questions, to receive information and reassurance and to express and share feelings in safety.

The task of preparation is difficult and emotionally demanding. There are good reasons for many parents' reluctance to share information about illness and death with their children. They are struggling to maintain some control in an uncertain situation, they do not know how to begin, they want to protect their children from pain and they are themselves grieving. Children also want to protect their parents, and unless we actively encourage their participation, they will often try to pretend that nothing is happening.

As external helpers we can begin by reassuring parents that we understand and share their concerns for their children. We can then gently explain that it is impossible not to communicate with children. They overhear conversations, they read the emotions and body language around them, they are aware of changes in routine. The issue is not whether to talk to them or not, but who will do the talking and how. Will the child receive confused and incomplete gossip, or consistent and regularly updated information from those who know and love him best, his parents.

The Environment

It is important to create an environment in the hospice, hospital or home that releases parents (and ourselves) from expectations that children should not be involved. We must invite their presence. Ward staff can brainstorm ideas which need not be expensive: displays of children's art in the foyer, some small chairs, a designated area, or box, for toys. Play, and drawing in particular, helps children act out their emotions and get them under control. Equipment might include plenty of paper and crayons, a doll in a bed and a medical kit. Videos and children's tapes can amuse both younger and older children quietly. The nurse should show parents and children the area by the bed where there is explicit permission for them to display their pictures, letters and cards. Not all children want to sit quietly by the bedside and some find conversation difficult. Older children might like to bring their homework in, some prefer to write rather than visit. Younger children might like to send in a home-made tape of a recited poem or the violin practice.

Information

Parents are often reassured by a reminder of the importance of answering children's questions as they surface, of letting the child set the pace. Children should not be pushed to talk nor frightened with excessive medical detail. Information needs to be clear, simple, truthful and repeated. It is helpful to start by linking explanations to things that children have already noticed. 'What have you noticed that is different about Mummy?' – 'She sleeps a lot and she hasn't got any hair'. We can then validate the child's experiences, assess their current understanding and correct any misapprehensions, always remembering to communicate feelings as well as facts. Information should be given gradually. 'Mummy is very ill. Mummy is so ill the doctors aren't sure they can make her better. Mummy is so ill that we can't make her better. Mummy is so ill that she is going to die'. We should not lie to children, nor make promises we cannot keep – 'We will make Mummy better'. A child in a frightening world will then have no-one to trust.

It is often helpful for a child to write out his questions (advance notice is reassuring for both parents and professionals) and to ask them with a parent, social worker and doctor or nurse present. Seven year old Mark whose father was dying from a brain tumour wanted to know:

- 'Can you stop the bad thing in Daddy's brain?'
- 'Can Daddy come home?'
- 'What will happen to Daddy's heart?'

It is important to remember that some explanations of death are confusing. 'Daddy has gone to sleep' can lead to the response, 'I shall stay awake all night'. Explanations should be simple and factual. 'When someone dies their body stops working'. The team need to be aware of the family's beliefs and careful not to conflict with them.

Reassurance

Children facing the death of a parent need reassurance about their own continuing care. Whether we raise it or not they will be wondering who will look after them, who will take them to school, who will come when they cry in the night. It is an enormous relief to them and their parents when these painful issues are addressed. Michael, aged 10, and Lucy, aged 6, had a meeting with the doctor, social worker, father, granny and dying mother. Their father talked about the nanny he was seeking, their mother voiced her approval and granny reassured them of her presence in the holidays. They also, very importantly, heard from their father about the things that would not change, that weekend swimming expeditions would continue.

Children need explicit reassurance that cancer is not contagious, that neither they nor other relatives are likely to become ill and die, that not all medicines make your hair fall out. Mark needed to know that it was his father's brain tumour that caused his short temper and aggression, not his own 'bad' behaviour.

Teenagers need special help. It is hard to lose a parent just at the point when you are trying to achieve your own separation. It can be helpful for teenagers to be given their own separate opportunity to talk about their concerns with the doctor. 'Why wasn't the cancer detected sooner? What does blockage mean?' They need help to voice their feelings of – 'What about me?' – and reassurance that their resentment of the disturbance to their life is normal.

The taboo against sharing adult grief with children needs to be broken. Children learn how to grieve healthily by observing others. They should be allowed to comfort as well as to be comforted and parents need reassurance that no harm will be done by crying in front of them: 'I'm crying because I'm sad that Daddy is so ill'. Although children need to share their parents' grief they can also be helped by others. We can encourage grieving parents to widen their child's support network by involving other adults close to them; teachers, relatives, youth club leaders, etc.

Parents may need help to anticipate and understand some of their children's altered behaviour in bereavement. A child's grief is often acted out in behaviour rather than words. Anger, for example, may be expressed through bedwetting or rudeness to a teacher. Nightmares, poor concentration and low tolerance of frustration are normal.

Expression of Feelings

It is important that the child's loss is acknowledged. They too need a chance to say goodbye, like the little girl who came to visit her dying father and left her toy rabbit with him 'to look after him'. It was later buried with him. In her bereavement she often mentioned her satisfaction at her special good-bye to her father.

Parents are often anxious about funerals and whether or not children should attend. We can help them give children information in advance so that the child can decide what he feels comfortable with. Children generally cope well with things they have been prepared for. 'A funeral is a time for everyone who cared about Daddy to get together to say good-bye. Daddy's body will be put in a special box called a coffin'. If children do not attend the funeral, they should be told what happened.

Children need to be involved in patient care as memories of helping will be important later on. The nurse can show them how to help with drinks or to water the flowers. All staff need to make a particular effort to introduce themselves to children and to explain what is going on. What is a syringe driver and how does it work? Most children are fascinated by simple mechanics and explanations help them to get a strange world under control. It may be helpful to make a 'scrapbook' for children to fill in and discuss with their parents as a less threatening way of beginning difficult conversations. 'Write down the names of the people helping to look after Mummy. Draw a picture of Mummy. Which bit of her is ill?'

A particularly distressing experience for staff occurs when a dying parent refuses to see their child. Grief can be overwhelming and some parents need to withdraw. They need help to express their anguish and our assurance that we do not find their actions 'unnatural'. Parents in this position can sometimes be encouraged to make a phone call to children, or will agree to receive a call on the trolley phone, or a letter. By contrast, other patients will want their parenting role reinforced. They may like to make story telling tapes for younger children to listen to at home and to discuss what gift they can leave behind for their child: a favourite necklace, a watch.

Parents are Colleagues

It is not our job to take over from parents. They know their own children best and it is vital that we approach them as colleagues. Many of them will not want us to be directly involved with their children but will welcome suggestions – 'Some parents find it helps if . . .' Parents want to discuss 'What shall we say if . . .?' They may appreciate lists of books to read with their children or leaflets on children's bereavement which enable them to gain some intellectual mastery over the situation.

In talking to children with their parents we can lead by example. Parents want to do what is best for their children and they learn very fast. Just being part of one direct conversation between a nurse and a child can help them feel brave enough to continue themselves. We also need to tell parents not to be too hard on themselves. It is normal to shout at children when you are under stress.

Staff Pain

Finally we must remember our own needs. Working with children facing the loss of a close relative involves us all in considerable emotional pain. The inter-disciplinary team need to share their feelings and support one another. We need to remind ourselves, as well as the parents we meet, that children are survivors. Given a little help, bereaved children can grow up to become happy and healthy individuals.

11

Having No Answer

Leonard Lunn

Zorba the Greek	Why do the young die? Why does anyone die, tell me?
Scholar	I don't know.
Zorba	What's the use of all your damn books? If they don't tell you that, what the hell do they tell you?
Scholar	They tell me about the agony of men who can't answer questions like yours.[1]

Writing this chapter has proved to be one of the most difficult things I have ever done in terms of getting started on a piece of work. I am not new to prevarications but this has been something different. On sharing the problem with a colleague he wisely suggested that the problem might be inherent in the subject matter and to state the problem might help me to break through the feeling of paralysis. He was right, like the scholar above I am having to go into print saying 'I don't know' and like Zorba I had been wondering what was the point of another 'damn book', albeit chapter, without answers.

And of course that is the problem for all of us who work with the dying and those who love them. We dare to go into a far country that borders on heaven and hell and learn a thousand different ways of saying 'I don't know' and learn to live with less than answers but hopefully more than an empty silence. Most of us I suspect are deeply afraid and secretly ashamed of feeling that we have no answer even though reflection tells us there are few to be had.

There is an agony in having no answer, not just for those who suffer but also for those who share the question and there can be an enormous loneliness in having to say 'I don't know' to those in pain.

The genius of the hospice inter-disciplinary ideal and the salvation of those of us who work with it is that we do not have to say 'I don't know' alone. We survive, in part, because we respond together. The major part of our answer is the massive combined response we call palliative care: a combined professionalism that includes symptom control, nursing care, counselling, spiritual provision with all of the other support services represented in this book and more. We do not attempt an explanation but it is a response that approximates to an answer. The totality of our response seems to provide an 'atmosphere' that *faces down* the questions and shows that spiritual and philosophical questions can be met in part through quite prosaic channels. This understanding of our shared and total response should help us to resist a professional hierarchy and a spiritual or intellectual snobbery. We know for example that the love of God can be mediated through an injection or by how a cup of tea is presented. The way in which a person is listened to and how thoroughly his questions are heard is certainly some kind of answer, an appropriate response gives value and significance to the questioner and the question. To stay with the impossible question is to stay with the pain which the person asking already knows is unanswerable – at least in Zorba's terms. It is the sharing of the question that is important and the inter-disciplinary team represents a special level of attempted empathy by its human as well as professional response.

It is both more effective and a survival mechanism not to stand alone with a response any more than we would leave the questioner isolated with the question. Then to find a thousand ways of saying 'I don't know' to the big 'why questions and responding, not in unison, but in some kind of inter-disciplinary disparate harmony.

Having no solution is not the same as having no response. Our fear of confronting the agony of those we seek to care for is usually about Zorba's demand for an explanation, a verbal reasoned answer to the ultimate questions of life. And like the questioner we know that is asking too much. But when we can ask ourselves not – 'what can I say?' but 'how can I respond?' then having no answer becomes more manageable and releases us to be with those in pain. That is with science and kindness, skill and courtesy, objectivity and shared humility, harmonised by an inter-disciplinary team into a response that is heard. It can be an untidy harmony and never unison but it seems to hang together in the end and I suspect that much more is heard than we think we say.

We all know the big 'why' questions are unanswerable in terms of definitive answers but our combined inter-disciplinary response can, and often does, bring meaning into inexplicable suffering. Agreeing with the patient who says 'it is so unfair' gives him some peace in his own answer and there is a curious sense of meaning in affirming meaninglessness. To respond 'life does seem so unfair' is to bring the search to where the patient is, whereas to look for, or seek, to impose some form of justice on his circumstances is to create more pain rather than less.

When a young mother screamed at me 'Why, why am I dying, I was eight when my mother died and I know what my children will have to face', she knew I couldn't answer. But she was asking for a response more profound than an answer. The counselling response of the social worker and nurses was more an exploration of her feelings with a permission to express them rather than a formulated answer – and certainly not any kind of explanation or solution. Yet because of what I represented she needed me to accept the question, to live with it and therefore to be with her. Having responded thus then part of her answer, because she was a Christian, had to be ritualised in prayer and sacrament. This process always reminds me of RS Thomas' poem 'In Church' describing a priest in church after everyone had left

> 'The bats resume
> Their business. The uneasiness of the pews
> Ceases. There is no other sound
> In the darkness but the sound of a man
> Breathing, testing his faith
> on emptiness, nailing his questions
> One by one to an untenanted cross.'[2]

This regularly happens in hospices, hospitals and wherever there is suffering and certainly not just to the Chaplain on the team. One of the prime functions of a chapel in such places is for private and shared anger, confusion and questioning, it is to have a target and a safe place in them to be expressed. This makes God a useful member of the inter-disciplinary team or for some the God they cannot believe exists, yet who can somehow be confronted.

Linked with a search for meaning are the questions that focus on the area of guilt, eg 'am I being punished?', 'what have I done to deserve this?', or 'can I put things right with God?'. These are all questions of people asking for some help on the journey of knowing themselves to be accepted. The background of the questioner and the context of the question will tell us how to respond. A specifically religious and ritualised response may be needed from a priest, a chat with a nurse may be more appropriate or the counselling skills of a social worker may be required. It is always informative to remember to whom the question is addressed, which may indicate the level and style of the response being requested. The patient in the bath who says to a nurse, 'Look at me, how can God allow what I've turned into?' is asking for something quite different from the one who asks to see the Chaplain in the privacy of his office. I will never forget the occasion when a doctor asked me to see a patient whom he said wanted to make a confession but who turned out to have in her estimation heard her confession himself, so she had no need of a chaplain. The doctor could hardly believe he had answered this request let alone pronounced an absolution.

There is literally a profound untidiness within the order of an inter-disciplinary team being available to deep human need.

This incident also illustrates that we need to help one another hear each other's questions so that non chaplaincy staff may have some confidence in responding to 'spiritual' questions. At the very least we give one another the courage to stay with the questioner and the question.

The specifically religious response to the question of guilt and forgiveness will be determined by what is appropriate for the person concerned and certainly 'I'll send for the Chaplain' is not usually the best immediate answer.

Recently an elderly patient at St Christopher's told one of the Chaplain's Assistants that she had sorted everything else out 'so now I want to put things right with God, what do I have to do?' This kind of direct question is more complex that it looks. Eventually it transpired that what this lady needed was something liturgical and ritualistic – a response that was not at all evident in her background. A visiting priest came (these requests nearly always come when I am on holiday) sprinkled holy water, anointed and prayed over her in a way that we would have hesitated to do but which met her need precisely. This example illustrates that many people need certain questions answered by ritual and symbol. Ancient words and practice have a power to respond to some of the deepest needs of those who suffer and when these occasions take place it is one of our most effective statements to have them attended by different members of the inter-disciplinary team. Anointing, laying on of hands, baptism, confirmation, holy communion, weddings and funerals can all be performed in a variety of ways that address the central questions of life. We all share their significance because they are sacraments for the living, some of whom may also be imminently dying. Sometimes it is not right, or possible, to intrude upon the answers that the dying find for themselves. They surely see and touch a deeper level of reality than those of us further back on the road and theirs is a special privilege with a necessary privacy to be guarded. Just as the pain and the questions are theirs so are what they receive in the way of answers.

Another range of questions is focused upon the hereafter – 'Is there a heaven and a hell?', 'what will it be like?' This is associated with the need for some continuity between this life and the possible next with such questions as 'will it make any difference when I've gone?', 'will I see my loved ones again?', 'will you miss me?'

The more religious issues in some of these questions are, like most issues of belief, very personal and as these questions are usually addressed to us directly as an individual regardless of profession they must be answered as such. Hesitancy and a healthy agnosticism at least regarding the details of the afterlife will give our responses an authenticity and authority that will empathise with the questioner's inevitable doubts. For example 'Well, the way I see it . . .', 'Mmm. I've never been quite sure but I think, I believe . . .', The Bible doesn't spell it all out but it seems to me. . . .' 'Yes, I do believe in heaven, I think it may well be like the Lake District in spring time.' Humour is not out of place with our own very serious convictions and our honesty is always more convincing than apparent dogmatic certainty. This makes the non chaplain response more welcome. The shorter, less formulated, response of the nurse for example is probably more comforting and true for people than that of the 'professional'.

What we believe is important, but somehow we have to test our convictions against our own dying. It is much easier to believe in a punitive God if we are not likely to be meeting Him face to face this week. And would we be so assured about going to Heaven if we were about to find out for sure? If we can be in touch with a measure of the reality which exists for our patients and families we shall then be offering a response that is effective long after our words are forgotten. One patient reported that the Chaplain didn't seem to know a lot about what heaven was like but that he had helped him to face death with a conviction that 'where he was going was OK'. Whatever disciplines we represent it is 'me, this person' that is the vital answer and authentic response while our words are very secondary.

The questions looking for continuity and reconciliation beyond death may be answered at a variety of levels and again according to our own beliefs and usually on a very personal one-to-one basis with the questioner. Much orthodox religious belief gives a clear 'yes' to many of the questions concerning whether recognisable personality survives and the possibility of reconciliation. Most people who ask these questions are not looking for detailed blueprints, rather they are searching for meaning and a hope that will sustain them in the crisis of death. They are not usually testing the particular professionalism of our discipline but rather probing our common humanity and seeking a strength that is unrelated to our clinical or other function. So in the face of having no answer or at best a partial one the inter-disciplinary team stand naked together. These particular questions are addressed to people not to professionals, although paradoxically our professionalism in our different disciplines will create the confidence to ask and engage with the painful questions that lurk in the dark.

Those with a formulated and practising faith or belief system, contrary to popular opinion, have particular problems with facing the ultimate questions. This is due to the pressure, both internal and sometimes external, to provide answers. I suspect that even a religious foundation or the presence of a Hospital Chaplain may provide as much pressure as support. Guilt at not having precise answers and a general unease at having one's beliefs challenged by experience can produce the fertile ground for growth but be disturbing nonetheless, not least because little Western religion allows for very much mystery, aspiring to knowing rather than believing. If there is a professional answerer of questions on a palliative care team, whether it be Chaplain or other guru figure, then his job is to unite his colleagues, releasing them from guilt at what may feel like shared ignorance to believe instead in a shared mystery.

Recently a visitor to St Christopher's came to see me and related how when he arrived he noticed through the Chapel windows that Snoopy, our hospice cat, was asleep on the altar. He said that he felt he had already learnt something important about our work before he came through the door. For me this was a reminder that the inter-disciplinary team is usually bigger than we think and also that wrestling with the ultimate questions is no excuse for taking ourselves too seriously.

References

[1]   KAZANTZAKIS, N. 1952. Zorba the Greek. Simon & Schuster, New York.
[2]   THOMAS, R. S. 1973. Selected Poems 1946–1968. Hart-Davis, McGibbon, London. p104.

12

Confusion and Sedation

Marie Murphy

Confusion is a common symptom in people who are terminally ill. In her introduction to this book Saunders speaks of our aim in this work . . . 'to enhance the quality of living and relationships when there is only a limited time left.' The period approaching a patient's death can be a time of growth and reconciliation for the patient and the family, a time for healing rifts and saying goodbye. If the dying person is confused this time may lose its meaning and become instead a time of great anguish and distress not only for the patient but also for the family and those involved in their care. Families may carry disturbing memories of their confused relative with them into bereavement and this may influence their ability to cope with life and loss in the future.

It is a challenge . . . and it is catching

The inter-professional experience in hospice is that managing confusion in the terminally ill poses an enormous challenge. It challenges us not just as skilled professionals but also as human beings. It raises several medical and ethical dilemmas which cause us to question repeatedly our management approach. Confusion is also contagious. Caring for such patients can often lead to confusion within the team. The aims and expectations of management become blurred and confusion abounds.

Confused patients and their families need care in a secure and stable environment. The caring team need a confident and united approach . . . otherwise the patients will become more muddled and the situation becomes self perpetuating.

What is confusion?

Confusion means different things to different people. It is useful therefore to begin with the definition in Butterworths Medical Dictionary:

Confusion is defined as a mental state characterised by disorientation regarding time, place and person causing bewilderment, perplexity, lack of orderly thought, and inability to choose or act decisively. It is usually symptomatic of an organic mental disorder, but may accompany severe emotional stress and various psychological disorders.

Many people may demonstrate bizarre behaviour or be unable to think or act decisively but it is the simultaneous presence of disorientation that marks these features of confusion.

What does it feel like to be confused?

A model first used in the study of schizophrenia is helpful in understanding what it feels like to be confused. It is proposed that our awareness is made up of stimuli from our environment, our sub-conscious and our bodily sensations. A filter controls entry of stimuli into our awareness and normally it is possible to determine the source of a stimulus and to choose which stimuli to attend to, e.g.: focus on a flower ignoring surrounding birdsong or attend to a full bladder.

In confused patients it is proposed that the filter control-ling input from the environment is thickened and they are cut off from their surroundings. In addition, confused patients have a heightened awareness of their inner world and bodily sensations and they may misinterpret events occurring round them and become frighteningly aware of their heartbeat or material from their unconscious.

A typical example of this is an elderly man who is confused and in pain from urinary retention – he may suddenly become terrified as you approach the bed. The explanation for this is that he is in pain and unable to determine where the pain is coming from. He is under the misapprehension that you may be causing the pain and are now approaching to do more harm. Confused patients are often aware of their state but unable to do anything to improve things. They feel cut off from reality and out of control. This can cause them great distress which in itself may serve to heighten their confusion.

Cause – Is it important?

A confused patient may have many underlying reasons to explain his state. Some of these causes may be reversible and result in the restoration of mental lucidity. Determin-ing the patients previous mental state and contributing causes to confusion will help clarify the hopes and aims of treatment. Without this understanding it is not possible for a team of carers to manage the problem effectively and help the patient's family. It may also be important for the patient to know what is underlying their present state and our hopes for them. A patient's family will often be able to provide the most accurate account of the patient's recent mental state and also know of any new changes in medication.

Clinical examination is imperative and investigations may be important in determining the underlying cause. In practice confusion in patients who are terminally ill is often due to a combination of factors with some reversible features and some residual deficit in brain function.

Management of Confusion

Having established the cause of confusion – what next? If there are reversible factors underlying it then appropriate efforts should be made to correct them. The aim of treatment is to reduce the distress the confusion is causing to the patient and family and if possible restore the patient to mental lucidity.

Sedation – is it the answer?

In a team discussion about confusion as an inter-professional group, words like frustration, helplessness, inadequacy and urgency were used repeatedly. Confused patients engender in us a variety of different feelings and an urge to do something *now* to relieve the situation. So often this leads to the prescribing of sedative medication. This may be an appropriate treatment, at least initially, but it is not the only answer. Medication as treatment for confused patients should only be used as part of a broader plan.

General measures

Confused patients are cut off from reality and feel out of control. Therefore attempts should be made to get them back in touch with their surroundings to re-orientate them gently and explain to them what has been happening. Because confused patients misinterpret activity around them it is important to eliminate many external stimuli, e.g. it may be possible to provide a well lit, single room. Familiar faces are very reassuring and family members and as few carers as is practical should be involved. A daily newspaper, calendar and clock may be sufficient to re-orientate some mildly confused patients. Conversely, a malfunctioning hearing aid may be enough to cause some patients to lose their tenuous grasp on reality.

Emotional distress can be enough to cause confusion in some patients. In patients who are dying the reality may be too painful and they withdraw inside themselves in response. I recall an elderly man who was slowly deteriorating from carcinoma of prostate with bone metastases. He became quietly muddled with no obvious physical or metabolic cause. One day while exploring his insight and view of the future with him, he became quite lucid and told me that he found leaving his wife of 40 years 'unthinkable.' We could not take the reality away, sedation may have numbed the pain a little but he remained quietly confused until he died. I recall another gentleman with a brain tumour who was confused and deeply distressed about his elderly wife at home alone and her inability to cope. His mental state improved considerably when reassured by one of the nurses that we were keeping a close eye on his wife and would be there to support her throughout his illness and into the future.

Patients often become acutely confused in the days approaching their death. They recognise the implications of their weakening state and become very frightened. Often they feel that some disaster is happening around them, i.e. the place is being burnt down, someone is coming to kill them. In this situation it is wise not to contradict them directly but rather pick up the mood of their thoughts . . .' It sounds like something frightening is about to happen.' 'Yes' 'might that be to you?' 'Yes' . . . and in this way you may be able to discuss their fears with them and help to ease their distress and so relieve their anxiety. Simple and practical measures such as these may significantly improve the situation. Attempts to treat reversible factors can continue in conjunction. Many patients may remain 'happily muddled' with no evidence of underlying distress. However, many other patients will be agitated and distressed and may, in addition, in some instances be a danger to themselves and others.

Quietly muddled but distressed

These patients generally have some insight into their confusion and are distressed by their cognitive deficit.

Sometimes simple explanations of the underlying cause is all that is needed to defuse the situation: 'You're not going mad but your illness has caused you to feel this way.'

When these measures prove ineffective sedative medication may be useful. An ideal medication regime should be an oral dose of a non-sedating long acting drug, aiming to achieve a situation where the sedative medication lessens the patient's distress without causing undue drowsiness.

Agitated, restless and distressed

Some confused patients become very agitated and hyperactive. In this situation they may prove a danger both to themselves and those around them. There is an urgent need to contain the situation. Gentle coaxing and explanation may prove effective but very often these patients are 'out of reach.' They feel out of control and may respond to a firm authoritative approach. This is an emergency situation and will require use of sedative medications to eradicate the patient's fear and agitation. A limited number of well known drugs should be used and the dose titrated according to the patient's response and history of previous exposure to sedation. Small doses of sedation can exacerbate the feeling of loss of control so in general in an emergency situation higher rather than lower doses should be used.

Having contained the emergency one must then consider the underlying causes or precipating factors, and decide on appropriate further management. Sadly in some cases, particularly in pre-terminal confusion, the only means of containing the patient's distress may be by continuing to sedate them to a state of sleepfulness.

Ethical Dilemmas

Managing confused patients and their families can stretch a team to its limits. In most other symptoms in palliative medicine it is possible to involve the patient in the decision making – they can make an informed decision on the best course of management with our guidance. Confusion is different. Although some confused patients clearly have insight and are in a position to be involved in treatment decisions, the majority do not. The caring team and patient's family have together to decide the best treatment options. Sometimes this decision involves sedating a patient who is already quite frail with the known risk that they may then develop a chest infection by virtue of sleep and inactivity.

Confusion is a symptom and underlying it may be many factors, physical, emotional and spiritual. What will be clear from the preceding discussions is that attempts should always be made to explore these. An elderly man confused due to uraemia in association with carcinoma of prostate became increasingly agitated and paranoid. He was a practising Roman Catholic and had been visited on several occasions by the Chaplain. His family felt he wished to see the Priest again. The Chaplain was recalled and apparently heard the patient's confession. His agitation and paranoia immediately settled and he remained confused but peaceful until his death less than a week later. In practice, however, the team is often left with a situation where the patient remains distressed despite the best efforts of the various disciplines involved.

Sometimes, the distress and confusion is so great that it is impossible to develop any form of spiritual or psychological link. In these instances, sedation is used to lessen the patient's distress so that more effective communication can take place. It is very gratifying when this happens but as stated previously, it can be difficult to establish a sedating regime which allows the patient to have useful wakeful periods.

Analogies have been drawn between the use of sedatives and the use of analgesics for relief of physical pain. The dose of analgesic required is that which relieves the pain – if it renders the patient drowsy in the process this fact would not preclude its use for controlling the pain. Similarly, with sedative medication, they are used to relieve agitation and anguish and the dose required may also cause a patient to be drowsy. In this instance the symptom is the anguish and the sedative is the medication to relieve this, which may or may not result in drowsiness.

As a team caring for the patient one of the concepts we have found helpful is to assess, along with the family, whether a patient's waking time is of any value to them. Are they continually distressed and muddled when awake, or are there periods of time which they still enjoy? It may in some cases, particularly in the final few days of life, become obvious that a patient is only settled when sleeping. In this instance, following discussion with team members and the family, a decision is taken to continue regular sedation so that the patient is asleep for long periods of time. This is never an easy decision and one is conscious that by remaining in a sleeping state the patient may develop a pnuemonia and perhaps die sooner than might otherwise be expected. In Kennedy's guidelines on treatment of the terminally ill he states 'A doctor's obligation in treating the terminally ill is to make the patient comfortable, which includes easing his pain. If, to ease his pain, the doctor must take measures which may hasten death, this is permissible, provided the doctors' principal and primary aim is only relief of pain.'

Similarly, a dilemma arises when patients refuse medication. In an emergency situation one is legally covered to administer a sedative against a patient's wishes if they are deemed to be incapable of making an informed decision and are felt to be a danger to themselves and others.

Patients may not accept medication proffered, believing in their paranoia that the staff are trying to harm them. In general, it is unwise to conceal the medication, e.g. in food or drink because this may heighten the patient's mistrust if discovered. Firm coaxing by a trusted member of family or staff may suffice but if not, Kennedy in his guidelines again states that where a patient is deemed incompetent, his family can make treatment decisions on his behalf. If the decision of the family is not deemed to be in the patient's best interest, this can be overridden by the doctor involved.

While these guidelines are very helpful in theory . . . in

practice sedating patients who are terminally ill remains a very difficult issue. The patient is the primary concern but we need also to consider the needs of their families, the other patients in the ward and staff involved in their care.

It is our experience as an inter-disciplinary team that we are continually discussing such decisions. Understanding the causes and aims of treatment is a vital part of effective care. Communication between staff involved, the patient and his family on an ongoing basis can allay much of the fear and anger that may surround the situation. We are constantly learning from the patient and their families. We sometimes feel we got it right . . . we are often saddened that it has not worked out as hoped, and a retrospective look at our care of confused patients and their families often makes the next confusion problem easier to manage.

13

Requests for Euthanasia*

Cicely Saunders

Those who work as members of an active interdisciplinary team find that they are developing both sensitivity in listening and confidence in the support of the whole group in challenging situations.

At no time are these needed more than when patients say that they want to die. Such requests frequently come unexpectedly in one to one situations and need to be listened to with total attention, without argument or any shade of censure. People may use these words to convey very different messages and it is essential that the real meaning of the particular request is carefully elicited. The subject should be clarified as much as possible there and then together with the promise of further discussion and a request made for permission for it to be shared with the rest of the team. Such a request is rarely refused for the person who voices it has reached a place of distress that has to be shared.

---

*Euthanasia in the UK has come to mean an act taken deliberately to cause a patient's death. Other decisions discussed here are sometimes termed 'passive euthanasia' but on the whole this is a confusing and therefore unfortunate term.

Possible meanings may be summed up as 'let me die,' 'I want to die' and, more rarely, 'Kill me.' The response to each will be different and most of the members of the team are likely to be involved.

Let Me Die

'Let me die' is a request that any treatment that is designed to prolong life should now be discontinued. The patient is afraid of a continued existence with a quality of life that can no longer be faced. Many people today fear that they will inevitably find themselves involved with all the procedures of an Intensive Care Unit with little or no choice in the matter. Decisions concerning appropriate as compared with possible treatments need to be discussed with the patient and the family after due consideration by the professional team. They may also need reassurance that the medications or procedures being given are designed solely for symptom control and will make the time remaining easier but not longer. A competent patient can refuse any or all treatments but needs to be suitably informed and choices respected. Not every patient understands this. Any decision should be open to review, for people must also know that they are free to change their minds. Family members can only make decisions for an incompetent patient in their best interests (Kennedy 1984). A team may need to consider this issue at length both with and apart from the family. At no time should the sad phrase 'There is nothing more to be done' be used. Much treatment can be offered in symptom control and support and this may need to be spelled out more than once to the patient, the family and the staff.

There are other matters to be considered. The team needs to discover what it is that makes continued life so grievous, and this may emerge in a series of conversations with different team members. Patients ask different questions and discuss different issues with the various professions. It often helps to give some idea of the likely time span for, while we must recognize how difficult it is to be at all certain in this area, some people are contemplating living on for months when the reality may more likely be weeks or days only. To explain this may be sufficient to ease the weary expectations.

Pain, weakness and the humiliations of dependence can all be tackled. The first is obviously the easiest to obliterate but the nursing team can lift much dependence by the way they carry out all their caring. Someone who can no longer turn over in bed without help may find the procedure has happened almost unnoticed because of the way it has been done and the attentive listening that has accompanied it.

Reassurance and explanation about the likely nature of the final coming of death may well be needed if anxious fears are to be eased. Hospice patients in a bay may be helped by seeing how others have died, 'I just want to go off peaceful like that old lady over there' said one elderly woman with confidence that she too would have her last symptoms controlled and that she would not be left alone.

I Want to Die

'I want to die' expresses anguish that demands attentive and experienced listening. Once again, the team member must try to disentangle the reasons for this wish. It often arises when past treatment for distress has been inept and listening cursory. There is likely to be much past emotional pain that can only be guessed at. The doctor must analyse and treat symptoms and the nurse monitor the treatment but here the social worker or chaplain member of the team, both well used to negative feelings and even despair, may help the expression of such feelings. Much of their power to hurt may be dispelled as they are voiced but the worker may need help from discussion with other members of the team in handling what has been said. Sometimes it reveals a treatable depression and a trial of medication may be appropriate. More often, the realisation that there is a consistent readiness to go on visiting whatever is said will gradually bring a conviction of personal value to the patient. It is not possible to give a sense of purpose in living out their time to another person. They must, and frequently do, find this for themselves, but we can often help to ease the sense of worthlessness. A grossly changed body image, the anguish of leaving unfulfilled responsibilities, the hatred of a passive role after an active life, can be recognized for the burdens that they are and the amazing endurance and ability to come to terms with adversity possessed by most people can be fostered by a team member who is able to sit alongside with no answers to give. But that member will need support in their own search for meaning from the rest of the team afterwards. To keep coming in this way may be extremely difficult in the isolation of Home Care and some team discussion from time to time essential if the professional is to continue to give real presence as they go alone to the home visit.

Kill Me

The specific request 'Kill me' or 'My father should not wake up again' is still extremely uncommon in spite of all the (often confusing) attention of the media to this subject. The person concerned almost certainly knows that we cannot do this but they may not be sure. We need to give a clear answer and a definite stance of this kind gives its own security. Once again, the team member concerned must listen, showing that they recognize the desperation that has led to the stark request and which may stem from much past fear or a need to control. It may also come, very understandably, from a person in poorly treated pain. Once again, all that can be done in palliative treatment must be presented and the promise given that in no way will that come to an end or the patient be abandoned. Some people need reassuring that death itself comes easily when good care is available and the relief of pain may mean that the request fades away forgotten.

The doctor (or nurse) may not embark on any conduct with the primary intention of causing the patient's death (Kennedy 1984). They may, however, if the patient wishes, help them to be more sleepy, though not to the point of permanent coma. This must be clearly explained and discussed with the patient, the family and the team. The latter must be clear what they are doing and why, time the offer of drinks and nursing care to wakeful moments and be ready to review the situation at any time. Some of the few who make a request for active killing will refuse the help to be more sleepy but they must know the offer remains and that they are free to change their minds.

Very occasionally, there will be a series of confrontational requests from one or more members of a family. It must be clear that while their expressions of anger may help towards the resolution of differences, this may not come about and the team as a whole will need to share their feelings and experience the strength of a cohesive group, greater than the simple sum of its parts. In one recent episode that stands out for its rarity, the difference between individual and institutional ethics was clearly spelled out by the social worker as the group as a whole, meeting in a crowded room as an emergency, recognized the strength that a previously undiscussed consensus had given them. There was no question of argument or blame for the person making the demand (the patient, though emotionally distressed, was more ambivalent). Discharge and Home Care were arranged but after a short time at home the patient wished to return to the hospice and died without physical distress three weeks after the first confrontation. She did not come to terms with what was happening and the small nursing team who carried out all her care needed all the support of the rest of the team. Unable either legally or professionally to give her what she still requested from time to time, no one withdrew from the caring and listening that they could offer.

'All That is Proper and Necessary'

Those who work in hospice or palliative care have taken the stand described above and the legal basis for this is discussed by Kennedy (1984) and summed up by Devlin (1985) as follows:

'If the first purpose of medicine, the restoration of health, can no longer be achieved, there is still much for a doctor to do, and he is entitled to do all that is proper and necessary to relieve pain and suffering, even if the measures he takes may incidentally shorten life. This is not because there is a special defence for medical men but because no act is murder which does not cause death. We are not dealing here with the philosophical or technical cause, but with the commonsense cause. The cause of death is the illness or the injury, and the proper medical treatment that is administered and that has an incidental effect on determining the exact moment of death is not the cause of death in any sensible use of the term. But . . . no doctor, nor any man, no more in the case of the dying than of the healthy, has the right deliberately to cut the thread of life.'

This position protects many vulnerable people for whom any legal right to die would so easily become a presumed duty to die ('I am only a worthless burden now'). Hospice care was summed up many years ago by the writer, 'You matter because you are you, and you matter to the last moment of your life. We will do all we can not only to help you die peacefully but also to live until you die.' We would not judge those who choose their own way out but as a professional team we do not believe we should take the step of deliberately aiding such a decision. Nevertheless, patients are constantly sent home with sufficient drugs to cover considerable periods of time, as was the patient referred to above. Those who take a deliberate overdose are extremely few and far between. It is their decision and this consideration has to be set against any feeling of failure by the team concerned. Here the basic philosophy of the nature of persons and their freedom of choice is concerned with both the patient and the team and its interpretation in a professional and caring setting may lead to enlightening discussion.

The first two requests discussed above are far more common than the third, but each and every time they must be faced, shared and the patient concerned helped through their distress as well as possible. The use that they and families so often make of the time remaining and that might have been lost, is the positive aspect of the stand hospice workers take against a deliberate shortening of life.

At the same time, it must be understood that all steps will be taken to relieve physical and, as far as possible, mental distress. It is not common that medication for terminal pain or restlessness should in itself shorten life, but that is a risk that must sometimes be taken when there is no alternative. This is discussed in Chapter 5. An explanation of any injection that comes at or near the end must be given to the family and sometimes needs discussion with new or inexperienced members of the team. Devlin's summary is helpful here but nothing replaces the careful full team discussion that constitutes the support needed in these situations.

That the requests considered above are sometimes put to a hospice team is an indication of the patients' freedom to express what they may think are unacceptable feelings. The majority are resolved peacefully in the end but at no time is a full team more needed.

References

DEVLIN, P. (1985) *Easing the Passing – The trial of Dr. John Bodkin Adams*. The Bodley Head, London.

KENNEDY, IAN McC. (1984) The Treatment Relating to the Terminally Ill. In: Saunders, C. (Ed). *The Management of Terminal Malignant Disease* (2nd edition). Edward Arnold, London.

14

Other Ethical Dilemmas

Margaret Harris

'Every problem is not an ethical problem, and every ethical problem is not a dilemma' write Curtin and Flaherty (i) and, while definitions can become very tedious, it seems important at the start of such a section as this at least to attempt an explanation of what we mean by ethical. Lisson (ii) defines ethics as 'a systematic way of making value judgements on human actions'. He goes on to say that 'the term *systematic* differentiates ethics as a process of organised and reflective analysis as opposed to nonreflective intuition or gut feelings.' Rather less technically, ethics is seen to involve the making of non-technical value judgements where there is doubt about which decision to make, or the belief that others might evaluate the problem differently. (iii)

Downie and Calman (iv) further suggest that a distinction be made between ethics as moral or value judgements broadly conceived, and ethics as codes of morality narrowly conceived, and following their distinction I start with, as it were, a broad sweep: the question of resource allocation. This is a fundamental ethical (and, of course, political) issue of our times, and is pertinent to all areas of health care, and global in its dimensions. At our recent Fifth International Conference, Dr de Souza, Medical Director of a Hospice in

Bombay, India, commented on the criticism he sometimes encounters in a country where it is a struggle to provide even the minimum of health care to a population whose growth is exponential. He is asked how he can justify spending so many rupees on high quality care for so few people who will shortly die anyway, when hundreds in his country never even reach the age of five years because of the poverty of medical care. The contrasts in our own country may be less dramatic, but they are there, and we need an answer to critics who would challenge those of us who work in a field where, generally, there *are* enough staff to do the job properly.

I turn now to look at three more narrowly defined areas with ethical implications, which tax us as an interdisciplinary team: the question of accountability and responsibility; that of confidentiality, and finally a look at whose needs we are, or *should*, be meeting.

Accountability/Responsibility

This is, perhaps, a particularly controversial area in a setting where interdisciplinary team work is valued highly. It has been suggested (somewhat tongue in cheek) that the doctors and nurses make the decisions, while the social worker and the chaplain are called in to pick up the pieces. This statement is both unfair and untrue, but it highlights some pertinent questions: What weight is given to each discipline? Who is involved in the discussion and decision making? Who makes the final decision and thereby 'carries the can'? Different disciplines are paid different salaries: part of the reason for this rests with the level of responsibility that each carries. Can decisions be truly democratic if, in fact, one member of the group is ultimately accountable for the decision made? The question of sedation has already been addressed in Chapter 13: the doctor writes the prescription but it will almost certainly be the nurse who administers the drug. And what weight will social workers and clergy be given in such a debate? Do the different disciplines adequately heed the work being done with a patient in areas other than their own?

Confidentiality

The very nature of interdisciplinary team work raises particular issues of confidentiality. Is it either right or necessary that every member of the team knows everything that a patient or relative may share with individuals within that team? I was first initiated into the use of 'pink sheets' as a staff nurse at St Christopher's. At the back of the notes of every patient there are loose, blank sheets of paper (which happen to be pink) where any discipline may record any 'significant' conversation (s)he has had with the patient or family member. These are extremely helpful and a communication tool but are as well, open to abuse and the subject of debate. Sometimes there seems to be no problem. I was called on one occasion to see a patient whom the nursing staff described as being in some kind of 'spiritual distress'. It turned out that the lady concerned was burdened by a 'sin' she had committed years before. She confessed, together we prayed for forgiveness, and peace came. I was able to record that a burden had been lifted, but there was no need, and many would agree I had no right, to share the nature of the burden with anyone else. However, supposing the confession had involved another family member whose relationship with the patient was a current issue for the social worker? Supposing this bit of information was a significant 'missing piece' in a complex family history? Disclosure to another discipline might enhance the care of that patient and the family. Conversely, disclosure of information such as 'this patient has committed murder/ incest' could adversely affect the care received owing to fear or prejudice. In such a situation is it right that every member of the team involved knows, at the risk of negatively affecting care? Is it right that such information should be *withheld* from staff who have regular contact with the patient?

The very documentation of acquired information can be an ethical issue, it being all too easy to express an opinion in place of a fact. We describe patients as 'sweet' or 'cantankerous', thereby stereotyping them and possibly prejudicing others' opinions of them. Do we make adequate allowance for patients (or relatives or colleagues, for that matter) to change, to grow, and to move on from the place where they are when we first meet them? Or do we neatly box them in and categorise them? Should patients have access to their own notes and, if so, will/should this affect what we write in them and how we express it?

Whose Needs?

Many of the ethical dilemmas we encounter as a team require an answer to the question: Whose needs are we seeking to meet? This leads us, inevitably, to ask: Whose needs *should* we be meeting? Sometimes there is a conflict between the needs of patient and family, at other times it is between patient and staff. The whole area of truth telling falls in this section. Consider the patient, Mr K, who was admitted to St Christopher's having been told by his wife that it was a convalescent home where he would be able to recover from his viral infection of the brain (Mrs K's euphemism for a brain tumour). Mrs K was adamant that the truth be kept from her husband and had been reassured by the staff that they would not seek to inform Mr K of his true diagnosis, but that if he asked they would not lie to him. Mrs K made sure there was little opportunity for her husband to ask questions, always being with him and being so protective of him that it was extremely hard to have any conversation with him alone. On pursuing Mr K's medical history it was discovered that the particular type of tumour from which he was suffering was amenable to radiotherapy. However, to allow Mr K to make an informed choice about treatment he had to know the truth about his diagnosis. What course of action should be taken?

The situation becomes even more complicated when the patient is unconscious – or even dead. I remember an occasion when I was called to see the wife of a patient admitted that day. Mrs A was very grateful for the offer of spiritual care for herself and her husband who was very ill and drifting in and out of unconsciousness. She and I talked in a separate room and discussed the possibility of having Holy Communion at the bedside together. She was very thrilled by this and I suggested we go together to Mr A and share our plan with him. 'Oh no,' she protested, 'if you ask him, he'll say no.' I gently explained that I could not and would not force Holy Communion on anyone against their wishes, however important it seemed to her that he should have it. Reluctantly she agreed and when I spoke with Mr A he became very angry with me for speaking with his wife and refused any spiritual ministry at all. The following day was Sunday and the Chaplain was visiting the ward where Mr A now lay unconscious and close to death. Mrs A asked for a blessing for her husband. For her, this was terribly important, but we knew Mr A's express wishes from the previous day. Whose needs were paramount? Should we disregard the wishes of the patient once (s)he is unconscious, and apparently unaware, in order to satisfy the needs of the aware, those who will live to carry memories into the future? It is not my intention to give answers, but our solution on this occasion arose from a suggestion made by one of the consultants who happened to be on the ward at the time, thus emphasising the value of interdisciplinary discussion.

The questions raised above concern the unconscious but they lead on to questions concerning the dead. Does a deceased person have rights? What about the lady who was admitted to St Christopher's and whose biggest, single anxiety was her cat. She insisted it be put down as soon as she died as she could not trust anyone to look after it as she had done. Her husband, however, wanted to keep the cat alive, evoking as it did for him so many cherished memories of his wife. Whose needs do we heed? Is a 'white lie' to the wife about putting the cat down permissible, if the intention is, then, to meet the husband's needs once his wife has died? What about the Muslim lady whose children are Christians. She wants a Muslim funeral: they want a Christian one. How do we advise the family?

Let us not forget the fact that we, as staff, also have needs. Is it ever right to put our needs before those of the patient, when the two are in conflict? What about the patient who appears not to be imminently dying, but who chooses to 'turn her (his) face to the wall'? Has the staff any right to 'jolly along' such a patient, encouraging them to sit out in a chair, to attend the Day Centre? We may do so, persuading ourselves that it is for the patient's own good, but is it? Is it not more a case of meeting our own needs? It may be easier for, say, the doctors or chaplain to allow such a patient to let themselves go, than for the nurses who have to cope with the situation hour after hour, shift after shift. Such patients do sometimes respond very positively to a little gentle encouragement and are ultimately grateful for the pressure put on them. Others die much more quickly than anticipated, leaving some staff with feelings of guilt for having misjudged the situation. How do we make the right decision in each individual case? The importance of interdisciplinary discussion cannot be over-emphasised since each member of the team will have established a slightly different relationship with the patient and so will have different insights to bring to bear on the debate.

Another situation which raises the question of whose needs are we meeting is where a patient expresses anger over past treatment which is perceived to have been inadequate or incorrect. If the patient's anger is justified and (s)he wishes to take legal action against the offending party, where do/should the loyalties of the staff lie? Should the staff collude with the family or with their colleagues: whose side should they take? Or is there an alternative way out? A specific example of a rather similar dilemma has just recently presented itself at St Christopher's. A patient with a brain tumour came to us following surgery which involved the removal of a section of the cranium, which was not then replaced. As the tumour enlarged, so it grew out of the artificial foramen created in the skull, enclosed only by a layer of skin. Instead of dying relatively quickly and painlessly from internal pressure on the vital centres this patient had a slow, lingering death filled with all sorts of fantasies of her brain exploding, and faced each day in the mirror with a grotesque, misshapen head. The whole team needed to talk regularly about this person, as clearly it was distressing for those caring for her as it was for the patient herself. Ought our doctors to take this up with those responsible for the surgery? It will not help this patient, but it may help future ones. Or should we 'let sleeping dogs lie'?

Returning to the statement with which I began this section I remind readers that a dilemma is a choice between equally undesirable alternatives and as such there can be no definitive 'right' answers. The temptation is simply to end with a multitude of unanswered questions but this is neither helpful nor conclusive. Instead, acknowledging my debt to Rumbold (v) I set out a few very general guidelines which may assist us when we are faced with some of the difficult situations this work imposes on us.

- *A knowledge of the law as it relates to the area of debate*   The law is a blunt tool for a delicate task, but since we are subject to it, we need to know the boundaries within which our decisions must lie.
- *A framework*   This is provided by professional codes of ethics which aid in the interpretation of the law. These also have their limitations: they are professionally exclusive; they cover broad principles only, failing to incorporate attitudes such as 'compassion'; they suggest that professional ethics are somehow distinct from the rest of morality. Professionals may be *given* their ethical codes, but they inevitably bring with them also their own individual attitudes, beliefs and values to their professional work.

- *A knowledge and understanding of ethical issues*   We need to recognise the cultural influence on decision making and also to have some understanding of the different theoretical approaches to ethics. Our moral decisions may be less reasoned than we imagine, almost certainly being influenced unconsciously by schools of thought of which we have no formal knowledge.
- *A sound knowledge base*   This will prohibit the making of a purely emotional response. The facts of the situation must be known as fully as is possible, so that the decision reached is an informed one.
- *Honesty with and to oneself*   Shakespeare wrote 'To thine own self be true' and, when all is said and done, we have to live with the decision we have made and its consequences. This is a good principle but is perhaps less easily achievable in the team situation. Team work demands a level of humility and, at times, submission in its members and we need to be sensitive to and supportive of any member who is in a minority when an ethical decision is made.

Marx reminds us that philosophers have sought simply to understand the world, whereas the point is to change it, and Aristotle tells us that the end of the enquiry is not knowing but doing. Let us avoid the temptation simply to enjoy a good debate, but be challenged to look more closely at how we resolve, or attempt to resolve, ethical issues within the interdisciplinary team.

References

CURTIN, L. and FLAHERTY, M. (1982). *Nursing Ethics, Theories and Pragmatics*, p. 39. Robert J Brady Co, Maryland.

LISSON, E. L. (1987). Ethical Issues Related to Pain Control. In *Nursing Clinics of N. America*, **22** (3).

WULFF, ANDUR PEDERSEN, Rosenberg (1986). *Philosophy of Medicine*, p. 172. Blackwell Scientific Publications.

DOWNIE, R. S. and CALMAN, K. C. (1987). *Healthy Respect. Ethics in Health Care*, Faber & Faber Ltd.
RUMBOLD, G. (1986). *Ethics in Nursing Practice*. Bailliere Tyndall.
See KENNEDY, I. (1984). The Law relating to the treatment of the terminally ill. From *Management of Terminal Disease*. Edward Arnold.

Index